the intolerant gourmet

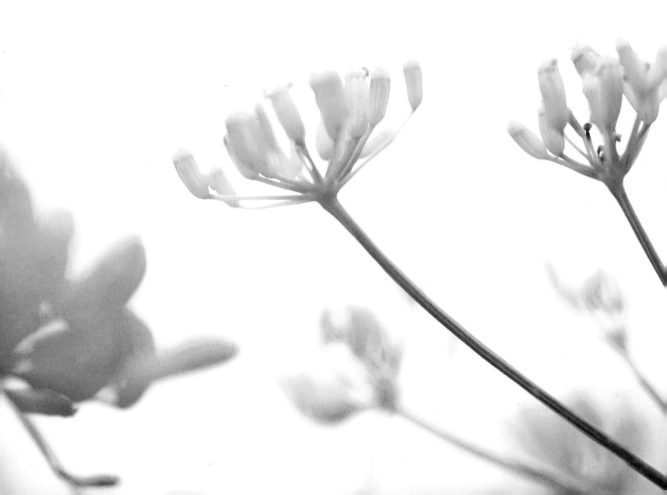

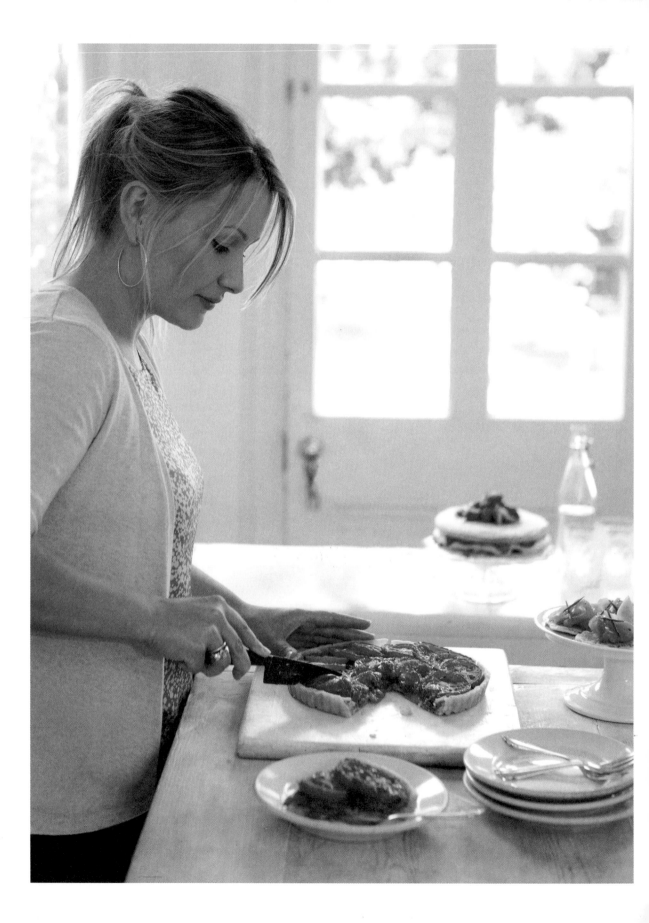

pippa kendrick
the *intolerant* gourmet

Collins

Contents

Summer

Autumn

Winter

Breads and Baking

Introduction

The Intolerant Gourmet is for everyone who loves food and who loves to cook. This includes anyone who suffers from an intolerance or allergy to certain foods, people not usually catered for by cookery books. For that reason all the recipes in this book are completely free from wheat, dairy produce, soya, eggs and yeast, and almost entirely free from gluten. Yet they taste fantastic – designed to inspire and make you want to eat. And, most important of all, they don't let on that there is anything missing. For this not an earnest cookbook but one that celebrates the joy of good food; every recipe could (and should) be served to friends and family, whether suffering from a food intolerance or not, without a single person finishing their meal feeling that they've gone without.

Through my own experience of learning how to cope with various food intolerances, I have met many fellow sufferers and this book has emerged as a result. *The Intolerant Gourmet* focuses on the culprit foods – how to avoid and replace the ones most commonly associated with food intolerances. It focuses less on full-blown food allergies, which are relatively rare and usually confined to one type of food, such as nuts or shellfish. By contrast, food intolerances are widespread and often multiple, with the sufferer developing a sensitivity to a whole range of foods. For this reason I haven't excluded nuts from this book as I find that, in the absence of other ingredients, they provide vital texture and flavour to my dishes. However, less than a third of the recipes contain nuts. Those that do are clearly marked and there is a wealth of choice for readers wishing to avoid them. For those who are allergic to any of the foodstuffs focused on in this book, such as wheat or dairy produce, then absolutely every recipe is open to you.

When first diagnosed with an intolerance or allergy, you may feel depressed at the idea of having to give up certain foods, but your diet need only be as restrictive as you make it. It takes a little extra forethought, admittedly, but within a short space of time preparing intolerance-friendly meals will become second nature. The benefits of avoiding the problem foods will leave you feeling so much better that you'll never want to go back to your old ways.

Cooking and eating are, by their very nature, sociable acts. Hence people who become restricted in their diet worry that they may also become restricted in their lives. Family meals or dinners with friends can become an act of isolation, with one meal for you and another for everyone else. Eating out can be equally fraught, its pleasures outweighed

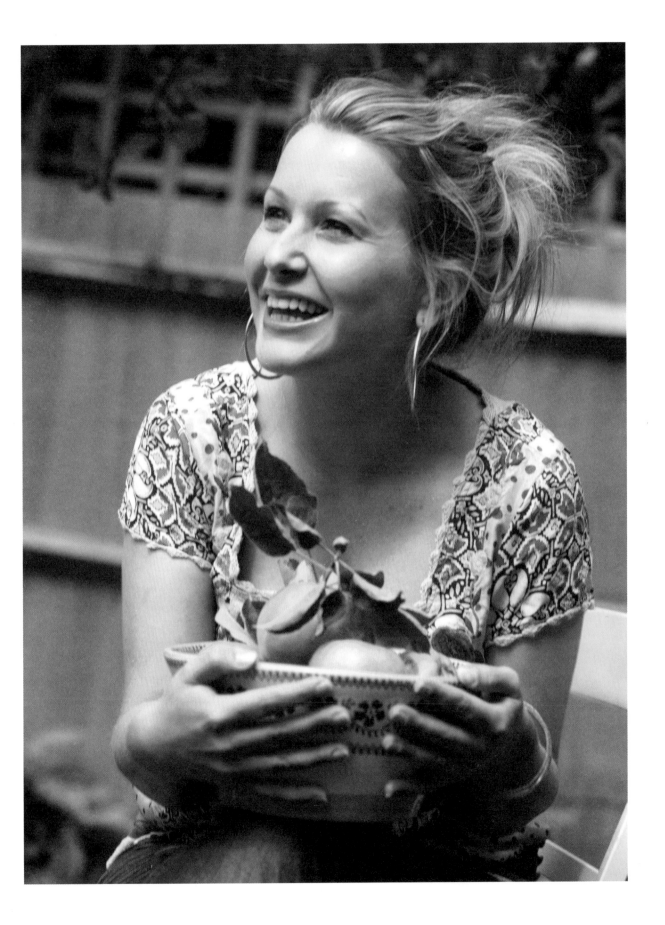

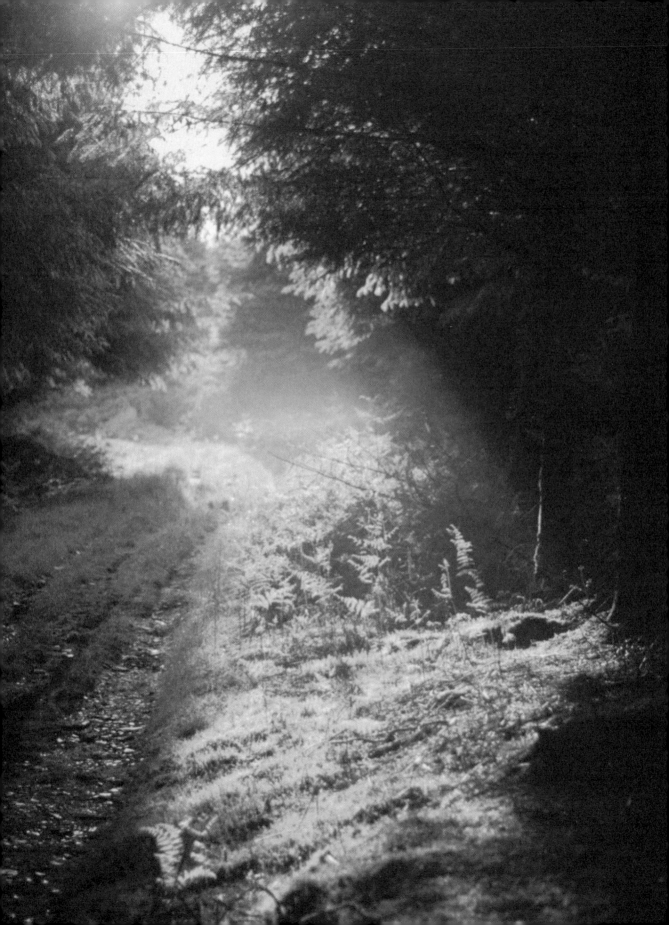

by the simple lack of anything on the menu that you can actually eat! Having lived with multiple food intolerances for years, I have experienced these frustrations many times. So when I began writing *The Intolerant Gourmet* it was very important to me that this was a cookbook that could be used by as many people as possible. In these pages you will find dishes that you can eat blissful in the knowledge that they contain nothing that could make you unwell. Not only that but they will make you and those eating with you feel both indulged and well fed. These are dishes that everyone can take pleasure in, whether they've a food sensitivity or not.

The recipes in this book aim not only to satisfy your dietary requirements, but also to inspire you in the way of intolerance-friendly home cooking. The thought of all the things you can't eat can seem overwhelming, but there are so many ways around this that you need never feel as though you are going without. Whether it is a combination of naturally non-allergenic ingredients, or an adaptation of a traditional dish using intolerance-friendly substitutes, these recipes will show you that being sensitive to certain foods does not mean a lifetime of deprivation. In fact, it can open up a whole new way of cooking that uses fresh ingredients, makes you feel fantastic and, most importantly, tastes really, really good.

The Intolerant Kitchen

The Intolerant Gourmet is all about the pleasure of eating – enjoying the delicious food you can have rather than craving the things you can't. But before delving into the recipes, it is worth defining what constitutes a food allergy and what a food intolerance and how they differ.

A food allergy generally causes an immediate allergic reaction, which triggers an immune-system response and severe symptoms. There is also such a thing as a delayed allergic reaction to food, as in coeliac disease, for instance, in which the sufferer is allergic to the gluten in wheat. Intolerance, on the other hand, is an adverse reaction to a particular food or ingredient that occurs every time the food is eaten, but especially if larger quantities of it are consumed. It is much more common than an allergy and, although far less dangerous, symptoms can be similar and it can be no less difficult to live with. Food intolerance occurs when the body is unable to deal with a particular type of food, such as wheat, dairy products or egg. This is usually due to a combination of factors – the body not being able to produce enough of the particular chemical or enzyme needed for the digestion of that food and an over-exposure to the food in question.

Food intolerance can be triggered by ill-health (following serious illness, for instance, or an operation on the digestive system), but in most cases it is brought on by an over-exposure to a particular food or foods. In Britain, for example, we consume a huge amount of wheat grain on a daily basis, without even being aware of it. It is quite normal for an individual to eat a wheat-based cereal for breakfast, a sandwich of some type for lunch, followed by a pasta-based meal for supper. The result is a disproportionate amount of wheat consumption in one day, and if this is repeated over time, it can easily lead to an intolerance to wheat.

Intolerances are rarely life-threatening, but they do cause very real symptoms, from bloating and abdominal pain to rashes, headaches and even depression. Such symptoms can begin hours or even days after taking the food in question, making it difficult to diagnose the cause. As a result, sufferers can find themselves living in a state where they never feel wholly well. Indeed, this may have gone on for so long that it will have become an accepted part of their lives. They can't remember a time when it was any better.

Once you have been diagnosed with a food allergy or intolerance, then you should of course try to avoid the problem food in all its guises. At the same time, it's important to build up your reserves of vitamins, minerals and essential nutrients and to support your immune system as much as possible. Avoiding the problem food needn't be a dismal business, however. You can buy a wide selection of products specially devised for sufferers from food intolerances and allergies, and some are worth their weight in gold in the kitchen. This cookbook uses a selection of the best, tried-and-tested products – for my list of recommended products and stockists, see pages 228–33. It also uses a range of allergen-free fresh produce to create recipes that are both rich in nutritional value and taste delicious.

Adopting an allergy- or intolerance-friendly diet does mean weaning yourself off all unnecessary processed and modified foods. When you can no longer rely on packets of biscuits or ready-made meals to fill a hole or provide an instant meal, learning to make the most of fresh wholefoods will make things much easier. Fruit, vegetables, pulses and meat – the foundation of good home cooking – are all intolerance-friendly foods, providing a great range of culinary options. The chapters in this book will encourage you to notice what's in season, too, so that you begin to make seasonal eating a natural part of your diet.

Foods for you

While it is easy to feel overwhelmed by all the foods you can't eat, it is far more helpful to concentrate on those you can. And the most important thing to begin with is to work out which of the staple foods you can eat and cook with in order to build up your intolerance-friendly storecupboard. Some will be familiar, while others may be new to you, but they'll soon become old friends. I've listed a tried-and-tested range of intolerance-friendly basics over the next few pages. All the foods listed are high quality and 100 per cent natural, with no artificial flavours, chemicals or preservatives. They are all widely available from health-food shops and big supermarkets.

Dairy-free milks

The dairy-free milks listed below are the perfect substitute for cow's milk in intolerance-friendly cooking. They are very useful in baking, and also create authentic-tasting custards and creams. You can make your own versions of the nut milks, but if you are buying them I recommend the varieties enriched with calcium, as every little helps!

Almond milk: a rich and creamy milk with a distinctive almond flavour, making it ideal for use in puddings and for pouring over cereal, especially granola or muesli. Most varieties come sweetened with agave syrup (see Products and Stockists, page 232) as it can be a little bitter without.
Hazelnut milk: a rich and creamy milk, with a distinct flavour of hazelnuts. Ideal for use in sweet baking and puddings.
Oat cream: a thicker, creamier version of oat milk, with added sugar and oil to emulsify it. It can be used in baking, to make ice cream and custards or simply to pour over puddings.
Oat milk: a creamy, savoury and ever-so-slightly grainy milk, this works very well in baking.
Quinoa milk: a thick milk with the distinctive flavour of quinoa.
Rice milk: a thin milk with a naturally sweet flavour. I use it on a daily basis, on cereal and as an accompaniment to tea and coffee. Rice milk heats well but will not froth or thicken when whisked.

Dairy-free fats and oils

There are a number of dairy-free margarines on the market, all varying in cookability and flavour. I recommend checking the ingredients carefully, buying only the trans-fat-free varieties (see Products and Stockists, page 229). Vegetable oils, being naturally dairy-free, are ideal for intolerance-friendly cooking.

Coconut oil: often called coconut butter, this is a hard oil (it sets at room temperature) that melts easily and has a distinctive, creamy taste. It is popular in intolerance-friendly baking as it reacts in much the same way as 'real' butter would do. Recently, it has received a lot of good press for its health benefits.

Flaxseed oil: an intense and rich oil. It is best used in small amounts – as part of a dressing, for instance, or drizzled lightly for an added nutritious boost – and should never be heated.

Groundnut oil: a light and flavourless oil. I would recommend this for frying and roasting.

Olive oil: an essential for any storecupboard. Olive oil is ideal for all savoury cooking and dressings and can be used in baking. I like to use extra-virgin olive oil for dressings and drizzling over dishes just before serving.

Rapeseed oil: a perfect oil for use in sweet baking as it has a fruity and slightly nutty flavour. It is very healthy too, being low in saturated fat and rich in omega 3, 6 and 9 oils.

Sesame oil: a strong and pungent oil. Most suited to Asian cookery and best used sparingly.

Sunflower oil: a good all-rounder, this has a neutral taste that makes it suitable for baking, roasting and frying.

Egg Substitutes

Replacing eggs in intolerance-friendly cooking can be a daunting prospect. Fortunately, there are a number of good 'egg replacers' on the market (see Products and Stockists, page 230). Consisting of natural starches and gums, they help to bind ingredients in baking, but without necessarily helping them to rise. For that reason I tend not to use an egg replacer in any recipe calling for more than two eggs, or I use it in combination with a little bicarbonate of soda. If you don't want to use commercial egg substitutes, there are a couple of other options available to you.

Apple purée: can be used as an egg substitute when making cakes, although it should be noted that it adds a distinctly fruity flavour to the mixture. You can buy apple purée from most health-food shops or from the baby-foods aisle in your supermarket. You can also easily make your own. Peel and core two small Bramley apples, chop into 1cm/½in cubes and combine with 2 tablespoons of apple juice or water. Cook over a low heat for around 6 minutes or until soft and then purée until smooth in a food processor or using a hand-held blender. Once made, the apple sauce will keep for up to 1 week in the fridge. To replace one egg in a recipe, use 2 rounded tablespoons of apple purée and ½ teaspoon of baking powder, adding the baking powder to the flour and the apple purée to the fat.

Ground flaxseeds: also known as ground linseeds, flaxseeds work well as a binder in intolerance-friendly baking, although they can create a gummy centre to whatever you are making. These are best for use in cakes, brownies, pancakes and biscuits. To replace one egg, my general rule of thumb is to use 2 tablespoons of ground flaxseeds and ⅛ teaspoon of baking powder blended with 3 tablespoons of water.

Gluten-free flours

Naturally gluten-free flours are far more prevalent than you may realise; it is the mixing of them that affects how successful they are in baking. You can buy some excellent pre-mixed varieties (as recommended in Products and Stockists, page 230), ideal for baking, but it's worth experimenting with your own mixtures too.

Buckwheat flour: a strong and 'earthy' flour, traditionally used for making blinis and soba noodles.

Gram flour: also known as chickpea flour. This golden flour has a distinctive nutty flavour and is widely used in Indian cookery, mostly for poppadoms and bhajis. It is great for coating patties and potato cakes before frying them.

Ground rice: more coarsely ground than rice flour, this is ideal for using in puddings and cakes as it gives a wonderfully light and airy texture to any mixture.

Masa harina: also known as corn or maize flour (not to be confused with cornstarch – see 'Baking Aids' page 20). This delicious golden flour has been used for centuries to make naturally gluten-free tortillas and

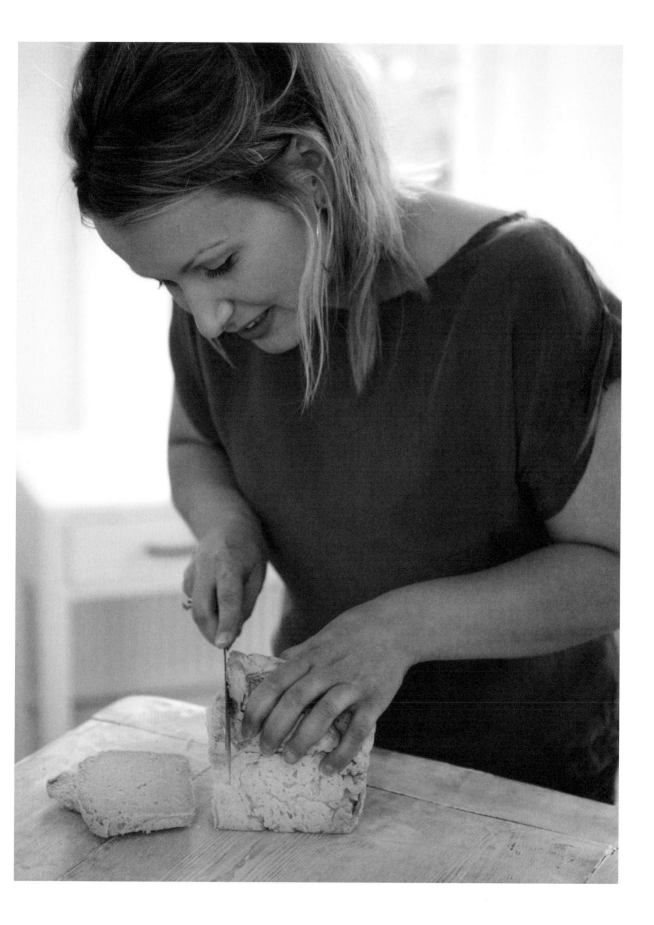

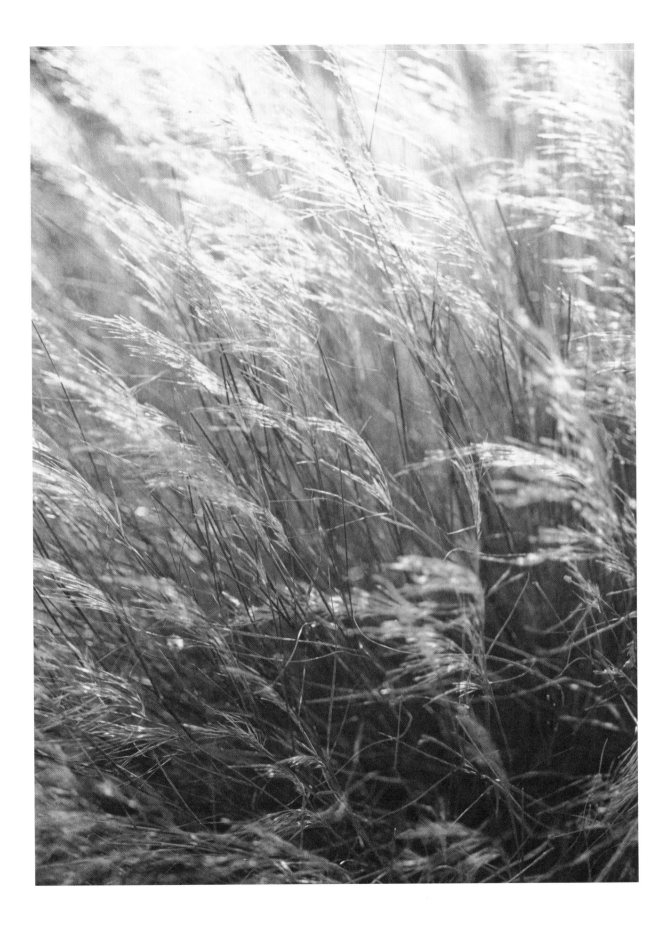

tamales. I recommend searching out a good-quality brand and experimenting with it; you'll find it well worth the effort.

Potato flour: a pure, white flour (not to be confused with potato starch), ideal for use in thickening sauces or as part of a blend with rice and quinoa flour for baking.

Quinoa flour: this flour has a strong and particular taste, making it unsuitable for some dishes. When combined with potato and rice flour, however, it makes a very good bread flour.

Rice flour: available in both its brown and white forms. Used as base for sauces or in shortbread, it has a slightly grainy texture that renders it unsuitable for use on its own in baking except when blended with potato and quinoa flour.

Rye flour: while containing no wheat, this flour is not entirely gluten-free and so is unsuitable for anyone trying to avoid gluten in all its forms. If you can tolerate rye then this heavy, dense flour makes a great sourdough loaf. It has a strong and distinctive flavour, making it unsuitable for sweet dishes, however.

Gluten-free grains

There is a common misconception that all grains contain wheat, but this is not so. There are an abundance of delicious grains that can replace wheat in a whole range of dishes.

Basmati rice, white and brown: ideal for use as an accompaniment to numerous dishes. Clean in flavour, basmati has the advantage of being quick to cook. I use it to stuff peppers and squash, in pilaffs and even to make rice pudding.

Brown rice, short-grain: a wonderful wholefood and natural detoxifier. Rich and nutty in flavour, it can be used as an accompaniment to many dishes and in place of white rice in risotto, paella and salads.

Buckwheat: not in fact a grain but a plant related to rhubarb. With a strong and earthy flavour, it can be used to make salads, while its flour is traditionally used for making pancakes and noodles.

Maize: otherwise known as polenta or corn, maize is a substantial grain that can be cooked with water or stock to produce a thick and creamy paste, or left to chill and then cut into slices and fried. Naturally golden in colour, it has a slightly sweet flavour, making it useful for baking cakes.

Millet: a strong-tasting grain often used in soups. It cooks in much the same way as rice and so can be used in any recipe where you would normally use rice.

Oats: a wheat-free food, oats can be tolerated by some coeliacs and gluten intolerants. Although oats contain a protein similar to that of gluten, it is the way that they are processed that really affects their gluten content. You can buy pure oats (meaning uncontaminated) that have been milled in a gluten-free environment, making them suitable for most gluten-free diets. The best gauge is to trust your instincts, listen to your body and avoid them if you feel that they have a negative effect.

Quinoa: actually a fruit rather than a grain, this can be used in much the same way as you would rice. Quinoa is both delicious and a great source of protein – I can't recommend it highly enough. With a slightly nutty texture, it benefits from the addition of stock or seasoning as it readily absorbs flavours.

Baking aids

All good baking requires some form of catalyst to help it leaven and cook well. With the removal of gluten, milk, butter and eggs from the list, it is really important that your remaining ingredients are up to the job! Using natural binders and thickeners is the way to go and there are lots of good-quality varieties on the market.

Arrowroot: a natural thickener. You can use it to thicken sauces and make glazes as it leaves a very clear sheen.

Baking powder: helps breads and cakes to rise. While generally gluten-free, it is always worth checking the label first – and to make certain that the brand you're buying is aluminium-free too.

Bicarbonate of soda: a natural leavening agent activated when it comes into contact with warm liquids. It is an ideal addition to intolerance-friendly cakes.

Cornflour: also known as cornstarch and based on maize (see page 19). It helps to thicken sauces and custards.

Xanthan gum: a plant gum that acts like the gluten found in wheat. Xanthan gum is the holy grail of allergy-friendly baking; it helps breads come together, pastry to roll and flatbreads to bend. It is the must-have staple of any allergy-friendly storecupboard.

Following the recipes

The recipes in this book are designed to work together – you can choose a selection of dishes from each section within one season and they will blend together to create a harmonious menu. When following the recipes, however, you'll need to bear in mind that allergy- and intolerance-friendly ingredients often don't work in the same way as their allergenic counterparts. For example, gluten-free flours are often far more absorbent than wheat flour and so require different quantities of liquids and fats to combine with them. Equally, using sunflower margarine as a replacement for butter is a useful and easy alternative, but margarine is simply a blend of vegetable oils and so when heated or over-whipped, its stability can change and affect the end result. When you cream the margarine and sugar in a baking recipe you should use a wooden spoon and lightly cream the mixture by hand, until incorporated. Beating the mixture too hard or for too long, and/or using an electric whisk, can cause the margarine to separate, which will result in an oily or 'fried' texture in your baking. The particular blends of flours and the other substitutes (whether milk, egg or butter) that I use have been specifically chosen, from personal trial and error, to create the best possible results. For that reason I would always recommend that you use the ingredients suggested as I cannot guarantee the same success if you use your own substitutions. That being said, experimentation certainly helped me, and so if you want to adapt the recipes using your own choice of ingredients, then go right ahead. Just be aware that you may have to adapt other parts of the recipe too.

Cooking notes

Fan oven temperature: if you have a fan oven, please reduce the temperature given in the recipe by 20°C/70°F.
Stocks: if not using homemade, please refer to Products and Stockists (page 233) for details of intolerance-friendly varieties of fresh stock, stock powder and stock cubes.
Teaspoon/tablespoon measures: 1 teaspoon = 5ml/⅕fl oz; 1 tablespoon = 15ml/½fl oz.

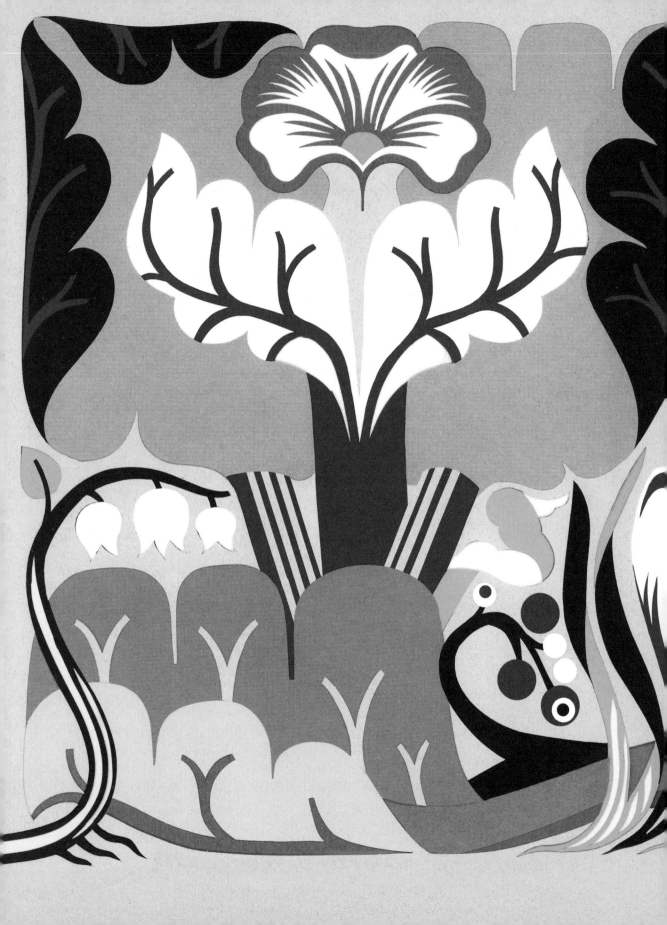

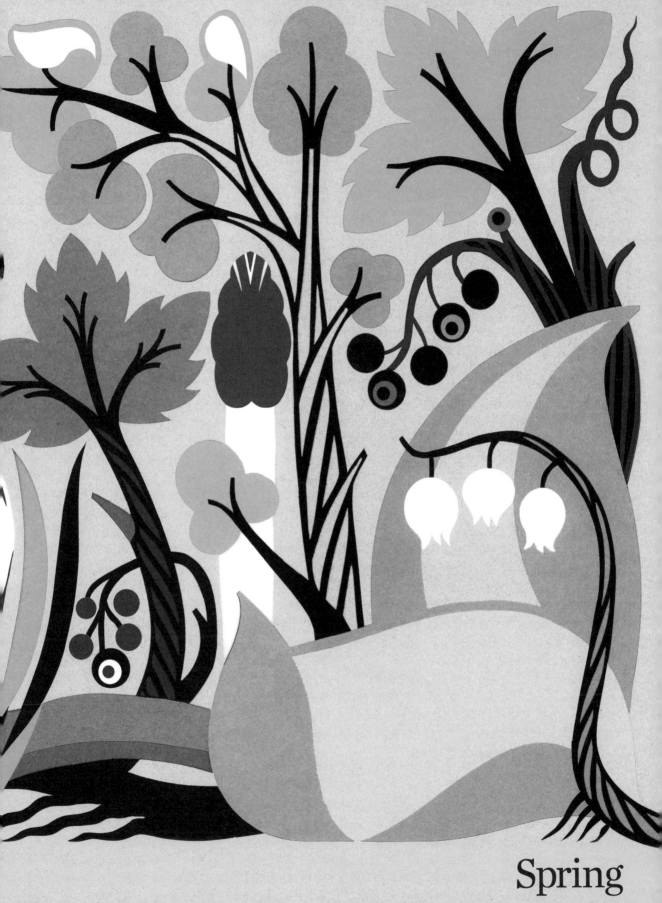

Spring

Spring imbues us with renewed energy and enthusiasm, and spring cooking should reflect this: we can say goodbye to the rich stews, hearty pies and warming soups of winter and reintroduce colour and crunch to our dishes. The Chicken, Watercress and Quinoa Salad (see page 34), for instance, offers a lemony zing and seasonal, peppery bite, while the Herbed Lamb on a Bed of Leeks and Cannellini Beans combines tender spring lamb with the mellow flavour of softened leeks to ring in the season (see page 43). The fresh, tangy theme carries through to the puddings: in the Rhubarb Streusel Tart (see page 58) the intense, sharp flavour of rhubarb is softened by the rich pastry and buttery, ginger crunch of the streusel topping. All the recipes in this section make the most of what's in season to embody this revitalising time of year.

Carrot and Coriander Soup

Serves 4–6

—

1½ tbsp olive oil
1 large onion
1 potato (unpeeled)
700g/1½lb carrots
1.2 litres/2 pints
  vegetable stock
A bunch of coriander
Juice of ½ orange
Sea salt and freshly
  ground black pepper

Soup is one of life's nurturers; it both sustains and comforts, warming one in body and soul, whatever the weather. For me, the best soups are the simplest: take some good-quality ingredients and cook them together slowly and you can't go wrong. This wonderfully vibrant soup is just the thing for a spring lunch; fruity and fragrant, and served with a slice of my Quinoa Bread (see page 217), it will brighten up any day.

Pour the olive oil into a large saucepan and place over a medium heat. Roughly chop the onion and add to the oil, cover with a lid and allow it to sweat for 4–5 minutes or until softened and beginning to turn translucent.

Chop the potato into 1cm/½in cubes and add to the onion. Cover again with the lid and cook for around 5 minutes, stirring frequently, until the potato has taken on a light sheen and is slightly softened.

Halve the carrots lengthways and chop into half-moon segments, then add to the potato and onion, season with salt and pepper and leave to cook for about 15 minutes, covered but stirring frequently, until the carrots and potato are tender.

Add the stock to the vegetables and bring to the boil, then reduce the heat to low and leave to simmer for 10 minutes.

Remove the soup from the heat and allow to cool down slightly. Finely chop the coriander and add it, along with the orange juice, to the soup. Using a hand-held blender or food processor, blitz the soup until smooth and velvety. Season with salt and pepper to taste, then heat through to serve.

Garden Soup

Serves 4

—

2 cloves of garlic
2 sticks of celery
1 leek
1 large red onion
2 carrots
1 potato
1 small sweet potato
1½ tbsp olive oil
1 courgette
100g/3½oz frozen peas
1.2 litres/2 pints chicken
or vegetable stock
A small bunch of
curly-leaf parsley or
watercress
Sea salt and freshly
ground black pepper

This soup is a variation on one of my mum's creations. So called because she always uses whatever is freshest and in greatest abundance in the garden, it manages to taste both rich and wonderfully fresh. My mum makes it with chicken stock (homemade, of course) for a satisfying, savoury depth of flavour, but you could use vegetable stock instead. And feel free to play around with whatever is in season: extra leeks, asparagus or spinach are all wonderful additions, although I would avoid adding any of the brassica variety (cabbage, sprouts, broccoli, etc.) as they tend to overpower. Serve hot with my Crusty White Loaf (see page 218), warmed through, for ultimate satisfaction.

Finely chop the garlic, celery, leek and onion. Peel the carrots, potato and sweet potato and dice into small chunks. Pour the olive oil into a large saucepan set over a medium heat, cover with a lid and sweat the onion, garlic, leek and celery for 4–5 minutes or until soft and translucent. Season well with salt and pepper, then add the carrots, potato and sweet potato and continue to sweat, with the lid on the pan, for a further 10 minutes or until they begin to soften.

Dice the courgette and add to the vegetables with the peas, then pour over the stock, cover again with the lid and bring to the boil. Once boiling, reduce the heat to low and simmer for 25 minutes.

Finely chop the parsley or watercress and stir into the soup. Remove from the heat and allow to cool for a few minutes, then, using a hand-held blender or food processor, blitz half of the soup, leaving the rest unpuréed for a chunky-textured finish. Season with salt and pepper to taste, then heat through to serve.

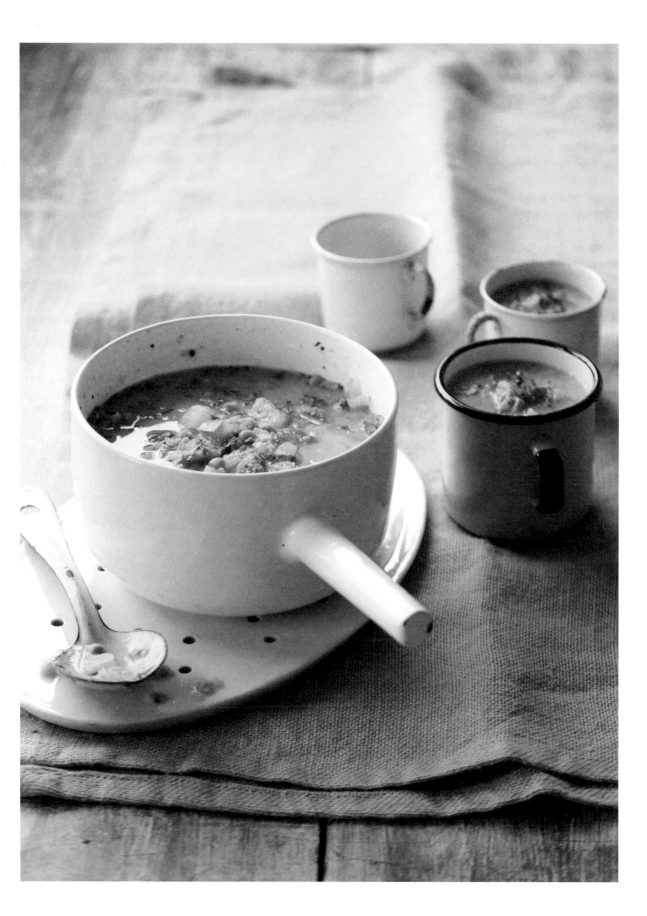

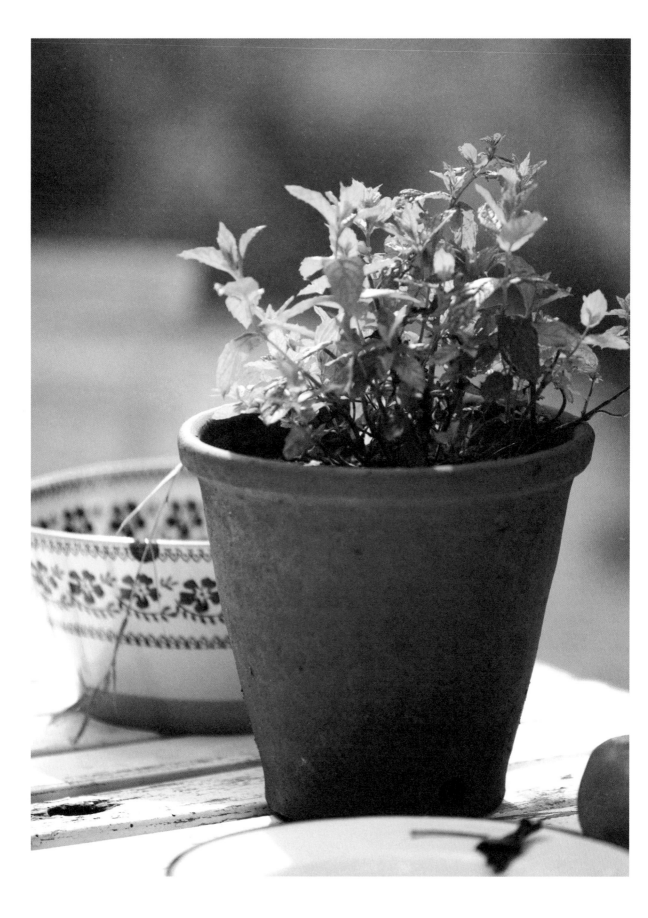

Warm Greek Salad sans Feta

Serves 4
Contains nuts
—

25g/1oz pine nuts
1 red onion
1 red pepper
1 yellow or orange pepper
1 large aubergine
1 clove of garlic
2 tbsp extra-virgin
   olive oil
1 tsp soft light brown
   sugar
½ cucumber
20 cherry tomatoes
15 pitted black olives
A bunch of mint
Juice of ½ lemon
Sea salt and freshly
   ground black pepper

This is one of my favourite salads – a lovely combination of bright colours and intense flavours. Here, the aubergine takes the place of the feta, its tender flesh melding with the sweetness of the peppers, the aroma of the mint and salty tang of the olives. I love to make this when friends come to visit – it's so simple to prepare but tastes quite complex and is really versatile. Served with a few green leaves and a slice of bread, it makes a refreshing light lunch, but it works equally well as an accompaniment to a larger meal. For a delicious supper menu, it would go wonderfully with my Spring Chicken with Lemon and Herbs and Roasted Sweet Potatoes (see page 42).

Preheat the oven to 200°C/400°F/gas mark 6.

Scatter the pine nuts on a baking tray and toast in the oven, turning occasionally to make sure they don't burn, for 5–6 minutes or until golden brown, then remove and set aside to cool.

Halve the onion, slicing it into thin half-moons, then deseed the peppers and cut lengthways into strips about 5mm/¼in thick. Trim the ends from the aubergine and cut into chunks approximately 2cm/¾in in size. Crush the garlic and place in a large roasting tin with the onion, peppers and aubergine. Drizzle over half the olive oil, tossing to combine, then sprinkle over the sugar and season with salt and pepper. Roast in the oven for 25–30 minutes or until all the vegetables are softened and browned around the edges.

Meanwhile, peel the cucumber and cut into 1cm/½in cubes, then halve the cherry tomatoes and black olives. Place in a large serving bowl with the roasted vegetables and mix together. Finely chop the mint and scatter over the salad, along with the toasted pine nuts. Pour over the remaining olive oil and the lemon juice, season with salt and pepper to taste and toss together so that the salad is thoroughly mixed and coated in the dressing. Serve while warm.

Prawn Noodle Rolls with Thai Dipping Sauce

Makes 12 noodle rolls
Contains nuts

—

110g/4oz cucumber
A small bunch of
    coriander
50g/1¾oz roasted and
    salted cashew nuts
100g/3½oz fine rice
    noodles
1 tsp toasted sesame oil
250g/9oz cooked and
    peeled prawns
12 spring roll wrappers
    (16cm/6½in
    in diameter)

For the dipping sauce
1cm/½in piece of
    root ginger
1 red chilli
A small bunch of
    coriander
1 tbsp soft light brown
    sugar
Juice of 2 limes
2 tsp toasted sesame oil
A pinch of sea salt

These little rolls are a beautifully packaged treat, perfect for a starter or served as part of a larger spread. They look and taste as though you have gone to a lot of effort but are in fact really simple to make. They have a light and clean flavour, while the combination of the rice noodles, sweet prawns, crunchy cashew nuts and cucumber provides a satisfying bite. The dipping sauce is a necessity and, if you wish, you can add a little to the filling of each roll before closing it. You can find spring roll wrappers in Asian stores or health food shops.

First prepare the dipping sauce. Peel and finely grate the root ginger, deseed the chilli and finely chop it and the coriander, then mix in a bowl with the remaining ingredients and 3 tablespoons of water. Cover and chill in the fridge until ready to use. (Left covered in the fridge, it will keep for 48 hours.)

Next peel the cucumber and cut into cubes about 5mm/¼in in size, finely chop the coriander and roughly chop the cashew nuts.

Cover the rice noodles in boiling water and leave for as long as instructed on the packet (usually around 10 minutes). Once soft and pliable, drain and place in a large bowl. Pour over the toasted sesame oil, then add the prawns, cucumber, coriander and cashew nuts and mix together until combined.

Prepare the spring roll wrappers by immersing each in cold water for a few seconds and then placing on a clean tea towel for 1 minute to allow it to soften.

Transfer each softened wrapper to a chopping board and spoon about 2 tablespoons of the rice noodles and prawns along the centre of the wrapper. Fold in two opposing sides of the wrapper and then fold over one of the remaining sides to cover the filling by about a third. Continue to roll the wrapper so that the filling is completely enclosed. Set aside on a plate and continue this process with each sheet of rice paper until you have made all of the noodle rolls.

You can then either serve the rolls immediately with the dipping sauce or cover and refrigerate for a few hours until ready to serve.

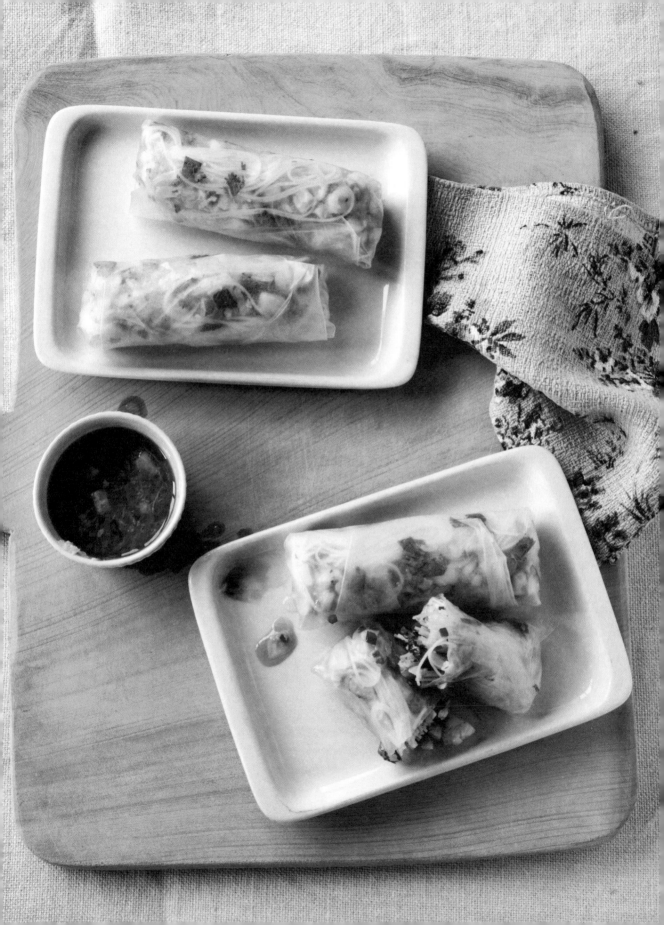

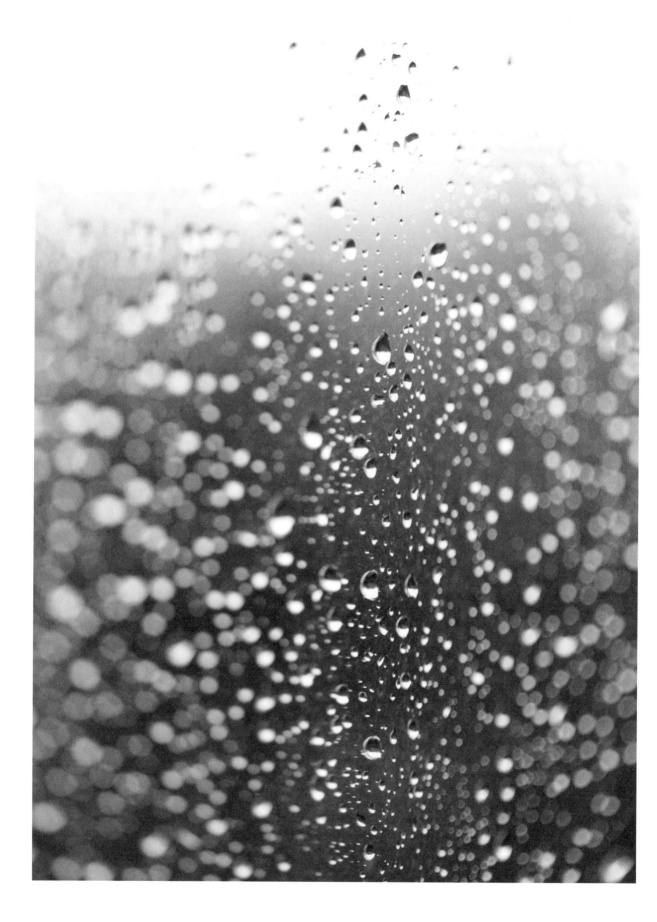

Falafel with Parsley and Tomato Salad

Serves 4

—

1 white onion

1 clove of garlic

1 x 400g tin of chickpeas, drained and rinsed

½ tsp sea salt

1 tsp ground coriander

1 tsp ground cumin

¼ tsp chilli powder

2 tbsp gluten-free plain flour (ideally Doves Farm)

2 tbsp groundnut or rapeseed oil

For the salad

A very large bunch of flat-leaf parsley

2 ripe tomatoes

½ red onion

1 tbsp extra-virgin olive oil

Sea salt and freshly ground black pepper

I simply adore falafel – dense, fragrant and completely moreish. A perfect treat when served as a starter, they are equally wonderful as part of a larger feast – my Honey-baked Leg of Lamb (see page 44) and Persian Jewelled Quinoa (see page 47) spring to mind. I like to serve them with a tomato and parsley salad – a variation on the Middle Eastern tradition of serving a bowlful of mixed fresh herbs with a meal. I think it lends the perfect bite and contrast to the softly spiced falafel. A dab of houmous wouldn't go amiss either.

Finely chop the onion and crush the garlic, then place in a food processor with the chickpeas, sea salt and spices and blitz until you have a rough paste. Tip the mixture into a bowl, cover and chill in the fridge for up to an hour or until firm.

Scoop up a tablespoonful of the chickpea mixture and, using the palms of your hands, carefully form it into a small round cake, approximately 2.5cm/1in in diameter. Repeat with the rest of the mixture to form about twelve falafel, then coat lightly and evenly in the flour and return to the fridge until ready to fry.

Next prepare the salad, first trimming the stalks from the parsley. Skin the tomatoes by placing them in a bowl, covering in boiling water and leaving for 1 minute. Drain and carefully peel away the tomato skins (they should slide off with ease), then slice in half, scoop out the seeds and finely dice the flesh. Dice the onion and combine in a bowl with the tomatoes and parsley leaves. Drizzle with the olive oil, season well with salt and pepper and toss lightly.

Heat the groundnut or rapeseed oil in a heavy-based frying pan and fry the falafel over a medium heat for about 3 minutes on each side or until golden all over – you may have to do this in two batches, depending on the size of your pan. Serve while hot with a handful of the fragrant parsley and tomato salad.

Chicken, Watercress and Quinoa Salad

Serves 4
Contains nuts

—

2 cloves of garlic
150g/5oz watercress
Grated zest of 1 lemon
    and juice of ½ lemon
175g/6oz quinoa
500ml/18fl oz chicken
    or vegetable stock
200g/7oz frozen peas
50g/1¾oz unsalted
    cashew nuts
350g/12oz cooked
    chicken
2 tbsp extra-virgin
    olive oil
Sea salt and freshly
    ground black pepper

This salad is light and crisp with a wonderful lemony, garlic zing. I love the combination of peppery watercress, succulent roast chicken and savoury quinoa. It is actually a very simple dish to create, especially if you are using leftover chicken, making it ideal to cook the day after roasting a chicken. You could even strip the meat from the chicken and then boil up the carcass with a few vegetables and a bouquet garni for some fabulous, homemade stock – perfect for using to cook the quinoa.

Peel the garlic and blitz in a food processor with the watercress and lemon zest until very finely chopped.

Place the quinoa in a saucepan and pour over the stock, then cover with a lid and bring to the boil. Once boiling, reduce the heat to its lowest temperature and leave to simmer very gently for 10 minutes. After 10 minutes, lift the lid and add the peas, then re-cover and cook for a further 5 minutes or until all of the stock has been absorbed by the quinoa. Remove from the heat and set aside to cool down.

In a heavy-based frying pan, dry-fry the cashew nuts over a medium–high heat for 3–4 minutes or until golden, shaking the pan regularly to ensure that they don't burn. Remove from the heat and season well with salt and pepper.

Next cut the chicken into small cubes, approximately 1cm/½in in size. Once the quinoa has cooled, fluff up with a fork and transfer to a large serving bowl. Gently stir in the watercress paste, add the chicken and cashew nuts, pour over the lemon juice and olive oil and season well with salt and pepper to taste. Toss thoroughly until well mixed and then serve.

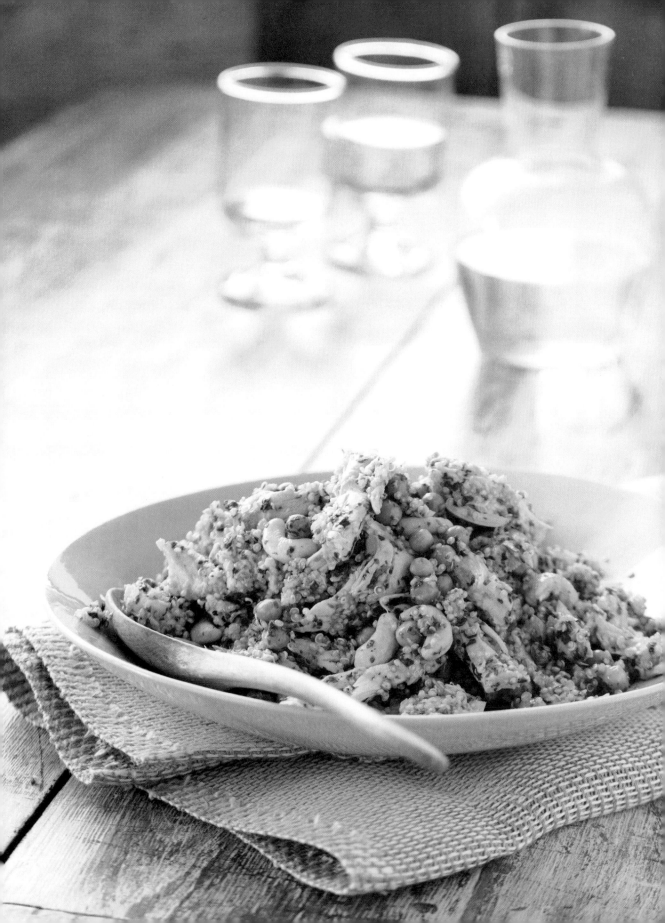

Chicken with Orange, Fennel and Olives

Serves 4

—

1 large red onion
2 fennel bulbs
2 cloves of garlic
A small bunch of
 curly-leaf parsley
3 tbsp olive oil
Grated zest of 1 orange
 and juice of ½ orange
4 skinless chicken breasts
100g/3½oz pitted black
 olives
Sea salt and freshly
 ground black pepper

I love the combination of oranges and olives – they seem made for one another, adding the kind of bright flavour to a dish that conjures up images of their sun-baked, Mediterranean origins. I recommend serving this with steamed white basmati rice, all the better to absorb the wonderful juices that pool around the roasted chicken and fennel. In addition to the rice, you could serve it with a green salad mixed with fresh herbs, although it would work equally well with wilted spinach or kale with perhaps a splash of garlic oil.

Preheat the oven to 200°C/400°F/gas mark 6.

First prepare the vegetables. Halve the onion and slice into thin half-moons, then trim the fennel bulbs and cut widthways into thin rounds. Crush the garlic and finely chop the parsley.

Combine 1 tablespoon of the olive oil and the orange juice in a bowl and season with salt and pepper. Using a sharp knife and cutting to a depth of 5mm/¼in, score each chicken breast diagonally three times (this will help the meat to cook evenly). Place in the orange marinade, stirring each breast in the mixture to ensure it is thoroughly coated, and set aside for at least 30 minutes.

In a large ovenproof dish or roasting tin, combine the onion, garlic, fennel, orange zest and olives with the remaining olive oil. Mix thoroughly, season well with salt and pepper and place in the oven to cook for 15 minutes.

Remove from the oven, stir well and then place the chicken breasts on top of the fennel and onions. Season lightly with salt and pepper and return to the oven to bake for 15 minutes or until the chicken is cooked through and, when pierced with a skewer, the juices run clear. Sprinkle with the chopped parsley and serve while hot, on a bed of white basmati rice.

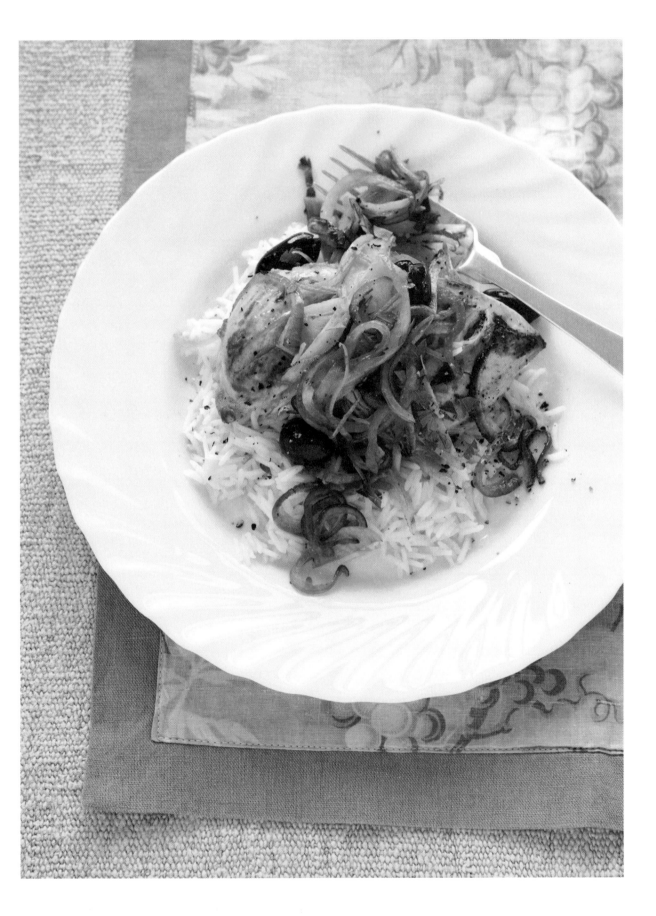

Chicken Rogan Josh

Serves 4
Contains nuts
—
6 skinless and boneless
    chicken thighs
2 red onions
3 cloves of garlic
1 red chilli (or more
    if you prefer)
2 large tomatoes
3 cardamom pods
2 tbsp groundnut or
    rapeseed oil
1 tsp chilli powder
2 tsp ground cumin
1 tbsp ground coriander
1 tsp turmeric
1 tsp ground ginger
1 tsp soft light brown
    sugar
A good pinch of sea salt
1 tbsp tomato purée
1 x 400g tin of chopped
    tomatoes
5 tbsp ground almonds
1 tsp garam masala
A small bunch of
    coriander

Rogan josh is one of those versatile curries that can be adapted to suit your palate. By that I mean that if you like your curries hot, rogan josh lends itself to the addition of a few extra chillies without losing any of its complexity of flavour. There is something reassuring about a sauce made of tomatoes and onions; it can really hold its own with a whole array of herbs and spices, while the ground almonds, when cooked, add a buttery note to the curry that enhances the whole dish.

Begin by cutting the chicken thighs widthways into slices about 1cm/½in thick. Halve the onions, slicing them into thin half-moons, crush the garlic and slice the chilli (or chillies) into fine rounds, keeping the seeds. Cut the tomatoes into quarters and crush the cardamom pods with the flat side of a knife.

Heat the groundnut or rapeseed oil in a heavy-based saucepan, add the onions and sauté gently over a medium heat for 5–6 minutes or until soft but not browned. Stir in the chilli powder, cumin, ground coriander, turmeric, ginger, sugar, crushed cardamom pods and salt. Cook the spices for a minute or two or until fragrant, then add the tomato purée, garlic and fresh chilli, and continue to sauté for a further 2–3 minutes.

Add the chicken and mix in thoroughly so that all the pieces are coated in the spice mixture. Pour over the chopped tomatoes, along with 150ml/5fl oz water, and add the tomato quarters. Cover with a lid, then bring to the boil, reduce the heat to low and simmer for 30 minutes or until the chicken is tender.

Once the curry is cooked, stir in the ground almonds and garam masala and simmer gently, uncovered, for about 5 minutes or until the sauce has thickened. Finely chop the coriander, sprinkle over the top of the rogan josh and serve with steamed white basmati rice.

Lemon and Cashew Nut Rice

Serves 4
Contains nuts
—

50g/1¾oz unsalted
 cashew nuts
½ tbsp groundnut
 or rapeseed oil
175g/6oz white basmati
 rice
½ tsp turmeric
A bunch of coriander
Grated zest and juice
 of 1 lemon
Sea salt and freshly
 ground black pepper

This mildly spiced rice is ideal for serving alongside any of the curries in this book. Indeed, it provides a fresh and zesty accompaniment to any Indian meal.

In a heavy-based frying pan, dry-fry the cashew nuts over a medium–high heat for 3–4 minutes or until golden, shaking the pan regularly to ensure they don't burn. Remove from the heat, season with salt and set aside to cool.

Pour the groundnut or rapeseed oil into a large saucepan and place over a medium heat. Add the rice and turmeric and gently fry for 1 minute, stirring continuously. Pour over 500ml/18fl oz water, cover with a lid and bring to the boil. Once boiling, reduce the heat to low and leave the rice to simmer for 10–15 minutes or until all of the water has been absorbed and the rice is fluffy.

Remove from the heat and leave to stand for a minute or two before fluffing up with a fork. Finely chop the coriander and stir into the rice with the toasted cashews, lemon juice and zest. Season with salt and pepper to taste and then serve.

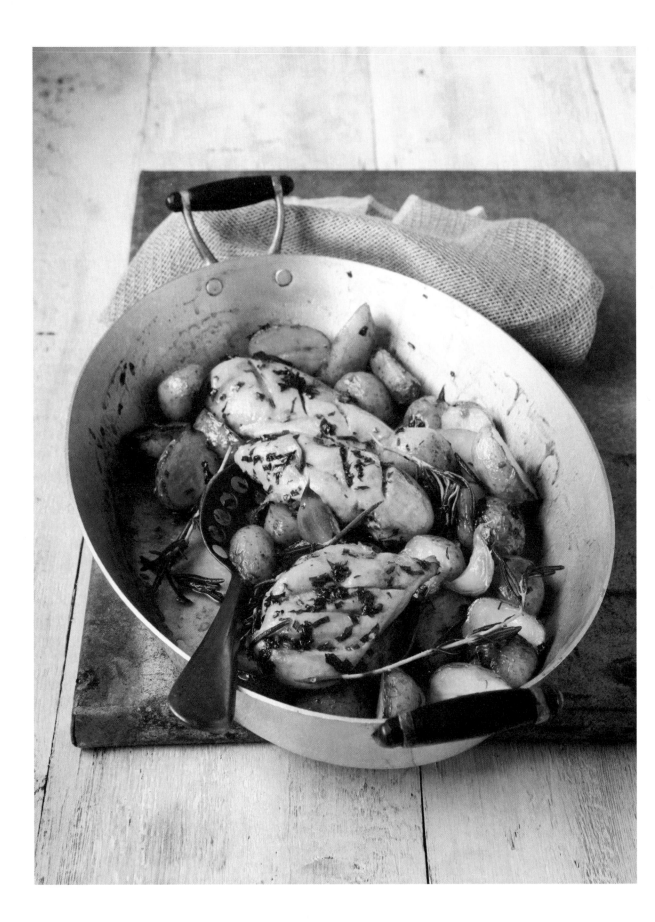

Roasted Redcurrant Chicken with Garlic and Rosemary New Potatoes

Serves 4

—

5 cloves of garlic
A small bunch of
   flat-leaf parsley
3 tbsp olive oil
2 tbsp redcurrant jelly
Grated zest of 1 lemon
   and 2 tbsp lemon juice
4 skinless chicken breasts
450g/1lb new potatoes
4 sprigs of rosemary
Sea salt and freshly
   ground black pepper

If I were to be scrupulously honest, I would say that this is really a cheat's version of a Sunday roast, with all of the flavour but half the work. It really is none the worse for it, however, and can transform a springtime supper or lunch into a time-saving delight for the senses. One of the beauties of this dish is that you cook it all together, not only bypassing the faff of having a numbers of pots and pans on the go, but also allowing the flavours of the dish to mesh in a beautifully fragrant way. Once the chicken is in the oven, you could lightly dress a fresh herb and baby-leaf salad to accompany it while sipping from a glass of something lovely – the perfect way to cook.

Crush just two of the cloves of garlic and finely chop the parsley, then add to a large bowl, mixing them with 1 tablespoon of the olive oil, the redcurrant jelly and lemon zest and juice.

Using a sharp knife and cutting to a depth of about 1cm/½in, score each chicken breast diagonally 3–4 times. Place the chicken in the bowl with the marinade, turning each breast in the mixture to ensure it is thoroughly coated and the marinade penetrates the cuts in the meat. Season well with salt and pepper, then cover the bowl and leave for a minimum of 30 minutes to absorb the flavours.

Preheat the oven to 220°C/425°F/gas mark 7.

Halve the potatoes and place in a large roasting tin with the remaining olive oil, whole garlic cloves and the sprigs of rosemary. Season well with salt and pepper and roast in the oven for 20–25 minutes.

Remove the potatoes from the oven and reduce the temperature to 200°C/400°F/gas mark 6. Place the chicken breasts in the roasting tin so that they are resting on top of the potatoes. Pour over the remaining marinade and return to the oven for 15 minutes or until the chicken is cooked through and tender. Remove from the oven, cover with foil and allow to rest for 5 minutes before serving.

Spring Chicken with Lemon and Herbs and Roasted Sweet Potatoes

Serves 4

—

1 x 1.6kg/3½lb chicken
1kg/2lb 3oz sweet
  potatoes
3 tbsp olive oil
Sea salt and freshly
  ground black pepper

For the herb rub
3 cloves of garlic
A small bunch of
  flat-leaf parsley
A small bunch of
  marjoram
Leaves from 4 sprigs
  of thyme
2 tbsp dairy-free
  margarine (ideally
  Pure Sunflower Spread)
Grated zest and juice of
  1 lemon (reserving the
  juiced halves) and finely
  chopped peel of
  ½ lemon
1 tbsp English mustard
  (1 heaped tbsp mustard
  powder mixed with
  1 tbsp water)
Sea salt and freshly
  ground black pepper

*This is a beautiful spring dish, simple to make but packed full of flavour.
I like to serve it with a large salad of fresh lettuce leaves: red oak, rocket,
cos and radicchio are all perfect. Equally, a pea and green bean salad
would make a great accompaniment.*

Preheat the oven to 240°C/475°F/gas mark 9.

Make the herb rub by first crushing the garlic and finely chopping
the parsley and marjoram. Mix them together in a bowl with the thyme
leaves, margarine, lemon zest and peel and mustard, seasoning well
with salt and pepper.

Using a spoon, carefully lift the skin of the chicken from around its
cavity and, with your hands, push the lemon and herb rub underneath
the skin, spreading over the chicken as far and as evenly as you can
without breaking the skin. Place the chicken in a large roasting tin,
stuffing the cavity with the leftover lemon halves, then pour the lemon
juice over the whole chicken and season well with salt and pepper.

Peel the sweet potatoes and cut into large chunks, approximately
5cm/2in in size. Surround the chicken with the sweet potatoes and
pour over the olive oil.

Place in the oven, immediately reducing the temperature to
220°C/425°F/gas mark 7, and roast for 1 hour and 10 minutes or until
the chicken is golden and, when pierced with a skewer, the juices run
clear. (Always test the meat of the thigh rather than the breast as it is
the slowest to cook.) If you feel the chicken or sweet potatoes are browning
too quickly, then cover with foil for the remaining cooking time.

Once roasted, remove from the oven, cover with foil and allow
to rest for 10 minutes before serving.

Herbed Lamb on a Bed of Leeks and Cannellini Beans

Serves 4

—

350g/12oz leeks
5 cloves of garlic
A small bunch of
   flat-leaf parsley
Leaves from 2 sprigs
   of rosemary
3 tbsp olive oil
4 lamb chops or 8 lamb
   cutlets
2 x 400g tins of cannellini
   beans, drained and
   rinsed
1 tsp soft light brown
   sugar
150ml/5fl oz chicken
   or vegetable stock
Sea salt and freshly
   ground black pepper

This recipe is perfect for spring, with all the wonderful fresh lamb that is available at this time of year. The ingredients are so simple, yet produce a classic combination of texture and flavour – the rich meat with the tender, tangy leeks and the creamy bite of the cannellini beans. This dish makes a meal in itself, but it's also delicious served with lightly crushed Jersey Royal new potatoes, drizzled with olive oil and sprinkled with sea salt.

Preheat the oven to 180°C/350°F/gas mark 4.

Halve the leeks lengthways and slice into thin half-moons, then crush the garlic and finely chop the parsley. Place the leeks in a large roasting tin or ovenproof dish, add the crushed garlic and the rosemary leaves and pour over the olive oil. Season well with salt and pepper and mix together thoroughly. Level out the leeks so that they form an even layer and then place the lamb chops or cutlets on top, spacing them evenly apart.

Cover loosely with foil and cook in the oven for 20 minutes, then remove from the oven and discard the foil. Scatter the cannellini beans over the leeks and gently mix together. Stir the sugar into the stock and pour over the lamb, leeks and beans, then return to the oven for 20–25 minutes or until the lamb is cooked through and tender.

Scatter the chopped parsley over a chopping board, then transfer the lamb chops or cutlets to the board, gently rolling the outside rim of each chop in the parsley to coat it. Serve the lamb resting on a large pile of the leeks and cannellini beans with the juices from the tin drizzled over.

Honey-baked Leg of Lamb

Serves 4

—

5 cloves of garlic
250ml/9fl oz oat cream, chilled
Juice of 1 lemon
1 tsp chilli flakes
2 tsp cumin seeds
1 tsp sea salt
1 tbsp olive oil
2 tbsp runny honey
1 x 1kg/2lb 3oz boned leg of lamb

This is such a glorious recipe, the lamb coated in a creamy spiced marinade that soaks into the meat and chars on cooking, producing the most divine combination of flavours. It's a great dish to serve friends and family as it looks so wonderfully generous placed on the table and carved for each person. You could serve it for a dinner party or as part of a more relaxed spread. The Persian Jewelled Quinoa (see page 47) lends just the right body and texture to the overall dish. Add a green salad and a large bowl of houmous and I, for one, am in heaven!

Preheat the oven to 220°C/425°F/gas mark 7.

Begin by crushing the garlic, then make the marinade by mixing this with the oat cream, lemon juice, chilli, cumin, sea salt, olive oil and honey. (It helps if the oat cream has been chilled first as it thickens up and acts like yoghurt.)

Lay the boned leg out flat, fat side down to begin with. Using a sharp knife, trim the lamb to make it level, scoring and cutting the joint if necessary, so that you end up with a flat piece of meat, reasonably even in thickness. Spread the marinade over both sides of the meat, working it into all the corners and cuts.

Lay the lamb on a rack in a large roasting tin and bake in the oven for 30–35 minutes. This will produce meat that is slightly pink in the middle, so cook it for an extra 5–10 minutes if you prefer it well done. The spiced cream will make a fragrant crust which may scorch during cooking, but don't worry as this only adds to the flavour.

Once cooked, remove from the oven, cover loosely with foil and allow to rest for 15 minutes, then slice into thick wedges and serve with the Persian Jewelled Quinoa (see page 47).

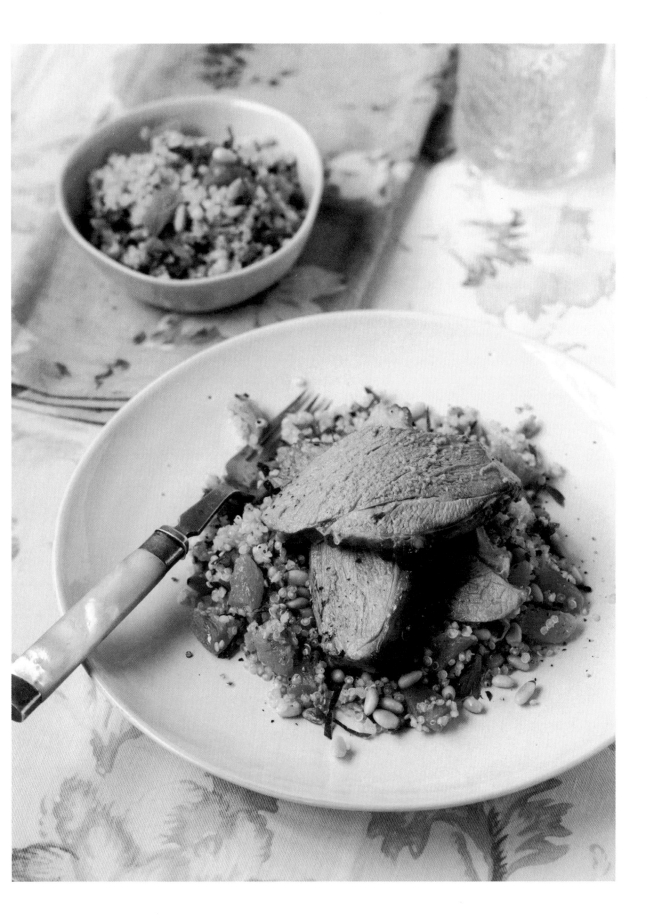

Chicken and Apricot Tagine

Serves 4
Contains nuts
—
30g/1¼oz pine nuts
2 red onions
150g/5oz soft dried
  apricots
A bunch of coriander
4 skinless chicken breasts
2 tbsp olive oil
1 tsp ground ginger
1 tsp turmeric
1 tsp ground cinnamon
425ml/15fl oz chicken
  or vegetable stock
Sea salt and freshly
  ground black pepper

*You will need a tagine
or heavy-based casserole
dish with a lid for this
recipe*

Like most spiced dishes, tagines benefit from being made the day before and then heated through the following day, allowing time for their flavour to develop properly. 'Tagine' refers both to the earthenware pot – a traditional north African cooking vessel with a distinctive conical lid – and to the food cooked in it, the spices and juices of the ingredients amalgamating to produce meat that is intensely flavoured and meltingly tender. If you don't possess a tagine, then a casserole dish with a fitted lid will do just as well.

Preheat the oven to 200°C/400°F/gas mark 6.

Scatter the pine nuts on a baking tray and toast in the oven, turning them occasionally to make sure they don't burn, for 5–6 minutes or until golden brown, then remove and set aside to cool.

Meanwhile, halve the onions, slicing them into thin half-moons, then halve the dried apricots and finely chop the coriander. Cut up the chicken breasts into 2.5cm/1in cubes.

Heat the olive oil in the tagine or casserole dish and gently fry the onions over a medium heat for 5–6 minutes or until softened but not browned. Turn the heat up slightly and add the spices and the diced chicken. Season with salt and pepper and stir to coat evenly, cooking for a minute or so before pouring over the stock.

Cover with a lid and bring to the boil, then transfer to the oven to cook for 15 minutes. Add the apricots and continue to cook for a further 10 minutes. Remove the lid and stir well, then return to the oven and continue to cook for another 5 minutes or until the chicken and the apricots are tender and the sauce has reduced to a thickened gravy. When ready to serve, sprinkle with the chopped coriander and toasted pine nuts before spooning on top of the Herb Quinoa (see opposite).

Persian Jewelled Quinoa

Serves 4
Contains nuts

—

50g/1¾oz pine nuts
50g/1¾oz golden
   sultanas or chopped
   dried apricots
175g/6oz quinoa
500ml/18fl oz vegetable
   stock
A bunch of coriander
A bunch of mint
Sea salt and freshly
   ground black pepper

So called for its Middle Eastern origins and the jewel-like, sweet sultanas it contains, this dish makes a delicious accompaniment to roasted meats or served cold as part of a selection of salads. I have used golden sultanas in this recipe but replacing them with dried apricots, chopped to roughly the same size as the sultanas, works equally well.

In a heavy-based frying pan, dry-fry the pine nuts over a medium–high heat for 3–4 minutes or until golden, shaking the pan regularly to ensure that they don't burn. Remove from the heat and allow to cool.

Cover the sultanas in boiling water and leave for 20 minutes – this will soften them and remove any yeast that may be on the outside. When softened, drain and set aside. If you are using apricots, then you don't need to soak them.

Place the quinoa in a large saucepan and pour over the stock, then cover with a lid and bring to the boil. Once boiling, reduce the heat to low and simmer gently for about 15 minutes or until the quinoa has absorbed all the stock.

Finely chop the coriander and mint. Using a fork, fluff up the cooked quinoa, then place in a large serving bowl, add all the remaining ingredients, season with salt and pepper and mix together.

Herb Quinoa

Serves 4

—

175g/6oz quinoa
500ml/18fl oz vegetable
   or chicken stock
A bunch of fresh
   coriander
A bunch of fresh parsley
Sea salt and freshly
   ground black pepper

Bursting with flavour, this dish is perfect for serving with the Chicken and Apricot Tagine (see opposite), but it also works equally well as an accompaniment to grilled meats or mixed with roasted vegetables. Feel free to use a combination of different herbs in this salad; almost anything works, except perhaps the woodier herbs such as rosemary and thyme.

Add the quinoa to a large saucepan and pour over the stock, then cover with a lid and bring to the boil. Once boiling, reduce the heat to low and simmer for about 15 minutes or until the stock has been completely absorbed.

While the quinoa is cooking, finely chop the fresh herbs and set aside. Fluff up the cooked quinoa with a fork and then add the chopped herbs, season with salt and pepper and mix together thoroughly. Serve while hot.

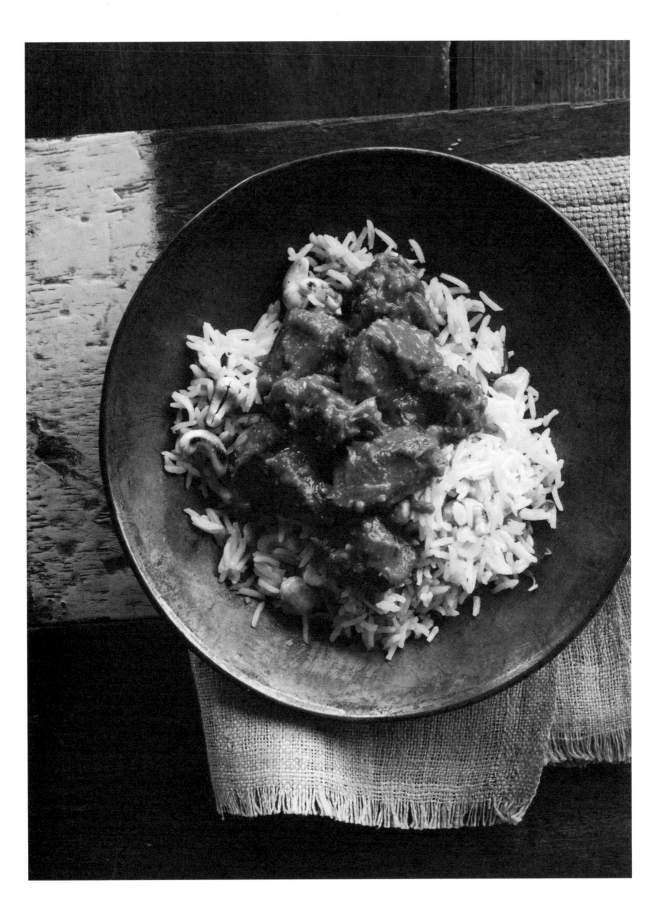

Lamb Korma

Serves 4
Contains nuts
—

4 cloves of garlic
2.5cm/1in piece of
   root ginger
2 white onions
3 cardamom pods
3 tbsp groundnut or
   rapeseed oil
2.5cm/1in cinnamon stick
2 bay leaves
1 tsp ground coriander
½ tsp turmeric
½ tsp chilli powder
2 tsp tomato purée
500g/1lb 2oz diced lamb,
   trimmed of excess fat
150ml/5fl oz oat cream
25g/1oz unsalted cashew
   nuts
A small bunch of
   coriander
Sea salt and freshly
   ground black pepper

This curry has a mild flavour and, although not heavy on the chilli, the blend of spices gives it a real intensity, while the ground cashew nuts produce an amazingly velvety and light sauce. I love the combination of lamb with this sauce, but chicken would work just as well. Equally, it really lends itself to being converted to a vegetarian version – potatoes or butternut squash with cauliflower, spinach and peas. Like all good curries, it is best made the day before so that the flavours have a chance to really develop. Simply heat through when you are ready to eat and add the fresh coriander to serve.

Crush the garlic and peel and finely grate the ginger, then mix together and set aside. Finely chop the onions and crush the cardamom pods with the flat side of a knife. Heat the groundnut or rapeseed oil in a large heavy-based saucepan, add the onion, cinnamon stick, cardamom and bay leaves and gently fry over a low heat for 8–10 minutes or until the onion is soft but not browned.

Add the ginger and garlic, along with the ground coriander, turmeric, chilli and tomato purée. Mix well and then continue to fry over a low heat for around 5 minutes, stirring occasionally. Add the lamb, season well with salt and pepper and mix together so that the lamb is fully coated in the spices. Pour in the oat cream and cover with a lid, then bring to the boil, reduce the heat to low and simmer gently for 30 minutes or until the lamb is tender.

Meanwhile, using a mortar and pestle, grind the cashew nuts with 2–4 tablespoons of water until you have a smooth and creamy paste. Once the lamb is cooked, scoop out the cinnamon stick and bay leaves and mix in the cashew paste, then raise the heat and simmer for a further couple of minutes. Roughly chop the coriander, stalks and all, and sprinkle over the korma ready to serve on a pile of Lemon and Cashew Nut Rice (see page 39).

Penne with Hot-smoked Salmon in a Garlic Cream Sauce

Serves 4

—

1 bulb of garlic
2 tbsp olive oil
250g/9oz hot-smoked salmon
A bunch of curly-leaf parsley
400g/14oz gluten-free penne
200g/7oz frozen peas
250ml/9fl oz oat cream
Grated zest of 1 lemon
Sea salt and freshly ground black pepper

Slow-roasting garlic cloves until they are tender, sweet and gooey is a sure-fire way to add glorious flavour to a dish. You can stir them into mashed potato, or spread them on warmed bread with a drizzle of olive oil. But I like them best stirred into a cream sauce, as in this recipe. The flavours of the hot-smoked salmon and garden peas mingle with the rich cream sauce, the garlic offset by the lemon zest, to make the perfect springtime supper dish.

Preheat the oven to 190°C/375°F/gas mark 5.

Peel away any loose papery skin from the outside of the garlic bulb, then slice off the top, about 5mm/¼in down from the tip, so that the inside of the bulb is left partially exposed. Place on a baking tray, chopped side up, pour over the olive oil and season lightly with salt and pepper.

Bake in the oven for 25 minutes or until the garlic cloves are soft and give when gently squeezed. Remove from the oven and allow to cool down slightly. When cool enough to handle, carefully squeeze out each clove from its casing and set aside.

Meanwhile, put a large saucepan of salted water on to boil. Peel the skin from the salmon and flake into small pieces. Finely chop the parsley and set aside. Once the water is boiling, add the penne to the pan and cook until al dente following the instructions on the packet – usually 10–12 minutes, depending on the brand of pasta. Add the peas to the water for the last 2 minutes of cooking.

Pour the oat cream into another large pan and add the roasted garlic cloves and lemon zest. Season well with salt and pepper and then whisk the mixture over a low heat until the garlic – which will be rich and gooey – is amalgamated into the sauce. Increase the heat so that the sauce begins to bubble lightly and continue to cook for 2 minutes or until heated through.

Drain the penne and peas and tip into the garlic cream sauce. Add the flaked salmon and continue to cook for a minute or two, stirring the mixture together very carefully and giving the pan a shake so that the pasta and sauce combine. Serve while hot, sprinkled with the chopped parsley.

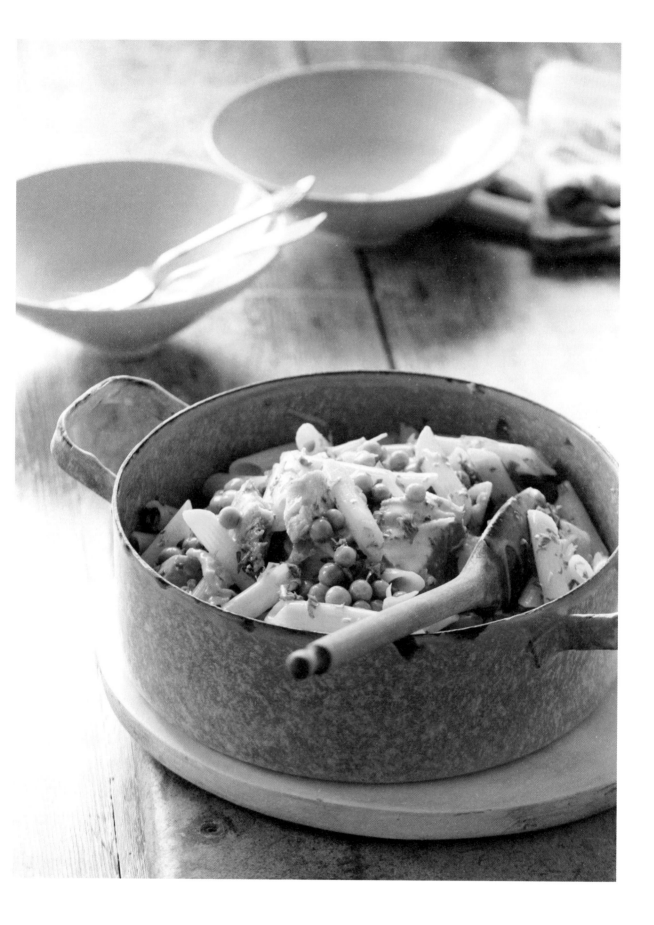

Spaghetti with Asparagus and Lemon Pesto

Serves 4
Contains nuts

—

400g/14oz gluten-free
   spaghetti
Sea salt

For the pesto
100g/3½oz pine nuts
200g/7oz asparagus
   spears
1 small clove of garlic
Grated zest of ½ lemon
5 tbsp extra-virgin
   olive oil, plus extra
   for drizzling
Sea salt and freshly
   ground black pepper

I have long thought that asparagus and lemon go gloriously well together. I like the way asparagus can hold its own among stronger flavours, its distinctive clean yet savoury taste allowing it to stand alone while still blending in with the crowd. This spaghetti dish is really just an extension of my love for homemade pesto. I've added a little lemon zest to the pesto to bring out the flavours and to offset the creamy taste and texture of the spaghetti.

In a heavy-based frying pan, dry-fry the pine nuts for the pesto over a medium–high heat for 3–4 minutes or until golden, shaking the pan regularly to ensure that they don't burn. Remove from the heat and allow to cool.

First snap off the woody ends of the asparagus by gently bending each spear between your fingers. The asparagus will start to give in one particular spot close to the base, allowing you to snap it easily at that point. Discard the woody ends and steam or boil the asparagus tips for about 4 minutes or until tender to the point of a knife. Refresh in cold, running water (to prevent further cooking) and set aside.

Meanwhile, bring a large saucepan of salted water to the boil, add the spaghetti and cook until al dente following the instructions on the packet – usually 10–12 minutes, depending on the brand of pasta.

While the spaghetti is cooking, make the pesto. Crush the garlic and then place the toasted pine nuts in a food processor and pulse until finely ground. Add the asparagus, lemon zest, garlic and olive oil, season well with salt and pepper and continue to pulse until you have a slightly rough paste. Season again to taste and set aside.

Once the spaghetti is cooked, drain and then return it to the pan. Tip in the fresh pesto and stir it into the hot spaghetti until it is fully coated. Drizzle with a little extra olive oil and serve.

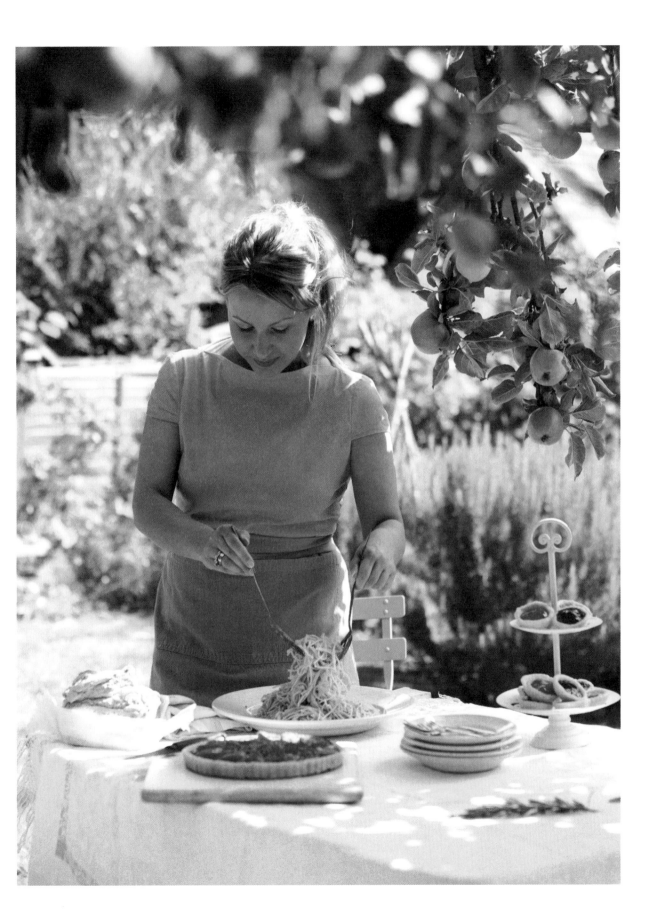

Sweet Potato and Spinach Curry

Serves 4
Contains nuts

—

1kg/2lb 3oz sweet
   potatoes
4 cloves of garlic
1 large onion
1 large tomato
1 red chilli
A bunch of coriander
3 tsp ground coriander
3 tsp turmeric
2 tsp ground cumin
3 tbsp groundnut or
   rapeseed oil
150ml/5fl oz vegetable
   stock
200ml/7fl oz coconut
   milk
100g/3½oz spinach
Sea salt and freshly
   ground black pepper

I truly adore vegetable curries. In many ways they are so much better than their meat counterparts, especially when you are cooking with starchy vegetables such as sweet potato, parsnip or squash. They have the ability to soak up all the intensity of flavour while providing a glorious texture at the same time. This curry is both warming and rich, made wholly comforting by the tender sweet potato, creamy coconut and tangy spinach. I recommend serving it with a bowl of steamed basmati rice, a salad of onion, coriander and tomatoes, some sliced bananas dressed in lemon juice and a few crisp poppadoms.

Preheat the oven to 200°C/400°F/gas mark 6.

Peel the sweet potatoes and chop into 4cm/1½in chunks. Crush the garlic and roughly chop the onion and tomato, then deseed the red chilli and finely chop both this and the fresh coriander.

Place the sweet potatoes in a large roasting tin, along with the ground spices and 2 tablespoons of the groundnut or rapeseed oil, season with salt and pepper and mix together until the sweet potatoes are well coated. Roast in the oven for 35–40 minutes, stirring occasionally, until the sweet potatoes are soft and tender and slightly caramelised at the edges.

While they are cooking, pour the remaining oil into a large saucepan, add the onion, garlic and chilli, and then fry on the lowest heat for 8–10 minutes or until softened but not browned.

Remove the sweet potatoes from the oven and add to the onion mixture in the pan. Pour over the vegetable stock and coconut milk and stir together gently. Add the spinach and chopped tomato to the curry, then cover the saucepan with a lid and bring to the boil. Once boiling, reduce the heat and simmer for 5 minutes or until the spinach has completely wilted. Taste, adding a little salt and pepper, if necessary, before serving.

Cauliflower and Chickpea Curry

Serves 4

—

2 cloves of garlic
2 red onions
4 large tomatoes
1 small cauliflower
1 red chilli
250g/9oz spinach
3 tbsp groundnut or
   rapeseed oil
1 tbsp cumin seeds
1 tbsp ground coriander
1 x 200g tin of chickpeas,
   drained and rinsed
300ml/½ pint coconut
   milk
1 tbsp garam masala
Sea salt and freshly
   ground black pepper

In this irresistible curry, the yielding texture of cauliflower mingles with the iron-rich tang of spinach, while chickpeas add body and bite to the dish, all enveloped in an aromatic coconut sauce. Perfect served with Lemon and Cashew Nut Rice (see page 39) and perhaps a poppadom or two.

Begin by finely chopping the garlic and onions. Place the tomatoes in a bowl, cover in boiling water and leave to stand for 1 minute, then drain and gently peel away the skins (they should slide off with ease) before chopping into quarters. Trim any excess stalk left on the base of the cauliflower and remove the outer leaves, then cut into small individual florets – no bigger than 3–5cm/1–2in in size. Finely chop the chilli, retaining the seeds, and set all the prepared vegetables aside.

Bring a large saucepan of water to the boil, then immerse the spinach and cook for 2 minutes. Drain and rinse the spinach briefly under cold, running water, lightly squeeze out any excess water from the leaves (taking care as they can be very hot) and then whiz to a coarse purée in a food processor or using a hand-held blender. Alternatively, you could chop the spinach by hand until very finely pulped.

Heat the groundnut or rapeseed oil in a large, heavy-based saucepan and add the onion, garlic, chilli, cumin seeds, ground coriander, chickpeas and a good pinch of salt. Sauté over a medium heat for 10 minutes or until the onion has softened but not browned. Add the cauliflower florets, tomatoes and coconut milk to the pan, cover with a lid and bring to the boil. Once boiling, reduce the heat to low and simmer gently for 30 minutes or until the cauliflower is tender to the point of a knife.

Stir in the puréed spinach and the garam masala, heat through for a couple of minutes, then season with salt and pepper to taste and serve.

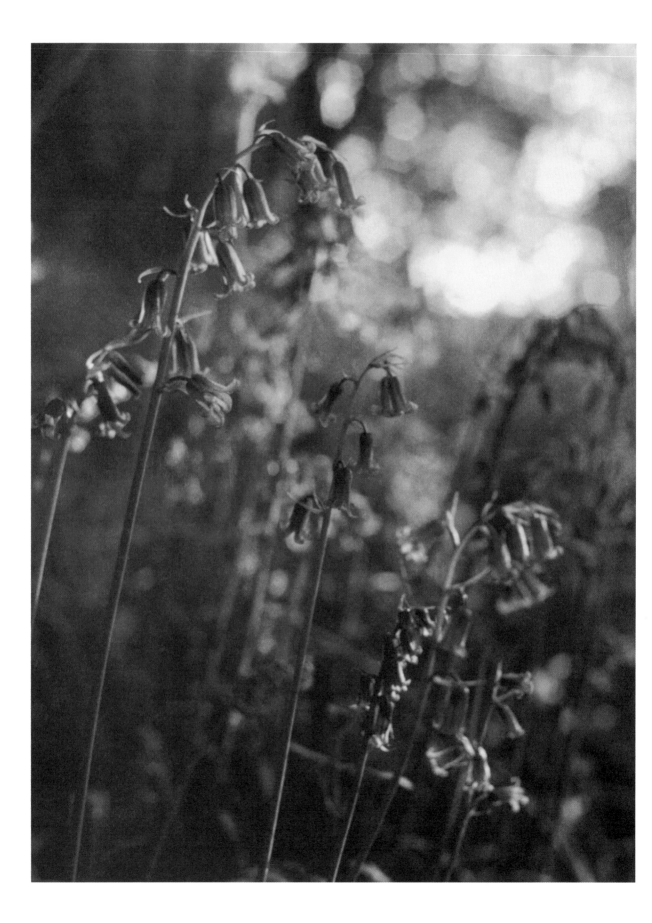

Spiced Spinach and Aubergine Stew

Serves 4

—

1 large onion
3 aubergines
3 tbsp olive oil
2 tsp cumin seeds
2 tsp coriander seeds
1 tsp smoked paprika
1 tsp ground cinnamon
100g/3½oz soft dried
    apricots
1 x 400g tin of chopped
    tomatoes
100g/3½oz baby-leaf
    spinach
Sea salt and freshly
    ground black pepper

This is a wonderfully fragrant dish, full of warming spices and complex flavours. I like to serve it with brown basmati rice and a good dollop of houmous. I have used baby-leaf spinach for this recipe as it is more delicately textured and flavoured; you can use the larger-leaf variety, but I would recommend that you remove any tough stalks and chop it roughly before adding to the aubergine and tomato.

Preheat the oven to 200°C/400°F/gas mark 6.

Finely chop the onion and dice the aubergines into 1cm/½in chunks. Place the diced aubergine in a roasting tin, cover with 2 tablespoons of the olive oil and roast in the oven for 25 minutes or until soft and golden.

While the aubergine is cooking, place the cumin and coriander seeds in a heavy-based frying pan and dry-fry over a medium heat for 2–3 minutes, shaking the pan regularly to ensure they don't burn, until lightly smoking and fragrant. Remove from the heat and grind to a coarse powder using a pestle and mortar. Alternatively, place in a plastic bag and use a rolling pin to crush them.

Heat the remaining oil in a large, heavy-based saucepan and fry the onion over a medium heat for 5–6 minutes or until soft but not browned. Add the freshly ground cumin and coriander, along with the paprika and cinnamon, and mix into the onion. Cut the apricots into quarters and add these and the roasted aubergine to the pan, then pour over the chopped tomatoes and stir to combine. Cover the pan with a lid and bring to the boil, then reduce the heat to low and simmer for 20 minutes.

Remove the lid from the pan, add the spinach and stir it in. Cook for a few more minutes until the spinach has completely wilted, then season with salt and pepper to taste and serve.

Rhubarb Streusel Tart

Serves 8

—

6 sticks of rhubarb
25g/1oz soft light brown
  sugar
1 quantity of sweet
  Shortcrust Pastry
  (see page 223)

For the streusel topping
75g/3oz gluten-free
  plain flour (ideally
  Doves Farm)
¼ tsp bicarbonate
  of soda
1½ tsp ground ginger
A small pinch of sea salt
75g/3oz soft light brown
  sugar
50g/1¾oz jumbo
  porridge oats
75g/3oz Pure Sunflower
  Spread (dairy-free
  margarine)

*You will need a 23cm/9in
tart tin with a removable
base for this recipe*

Glorious rhubarb, I am a fan of it in all its guises, whether in crumbles, pies or fools, but this streusel tart may just be my favourite. The biscuit base gives way to the tang of sweet-sharp rhubarb, while the streusel topping provides a buttery, oat crunch with a hint of warming ginger – a spice that just adores rhubarb. Serve warm with a scoop of Vanilla Ice Cream (see page 66).

Trim the rhubarb and cut into 1cm/½in rounds. Place in a large saucepan with the sugar, cover with a lid and cook over a low heat for about 10 minutes or until the rhubarb has softened and become gently stewed. Set aside to cool a little while you prepare the streusel topping.

Sift the flour, bicarbonate of soda, ground ginger and salt into a large bowl and stir in the sugar and oats. Add the margarine and, using your fingers, rub it in until the mixture forms soft, crumble-like clumps.

Preheat the oven to 190°C/375°F/gas mark 5.

Roll out the pastry and fill the tart tin following the instructions given in the Shortcrust Pastry recipe on page 223.

Using a slotted spoon so that any excess juice can drain away, spoon in the stewed rhubarb, spreading it evenly over the base of the tart and discarding the remaining liquid.

Crumble the streusel topping evenly over the tart, pressing down gently with your fingertips to fill any large gaps, then bake in the oven for 35–40 minutes or until the streusel is a deep gold and the pastry is cooked. Leave the tart in its tin on a wire rack to cool for 10 minutes before serving.

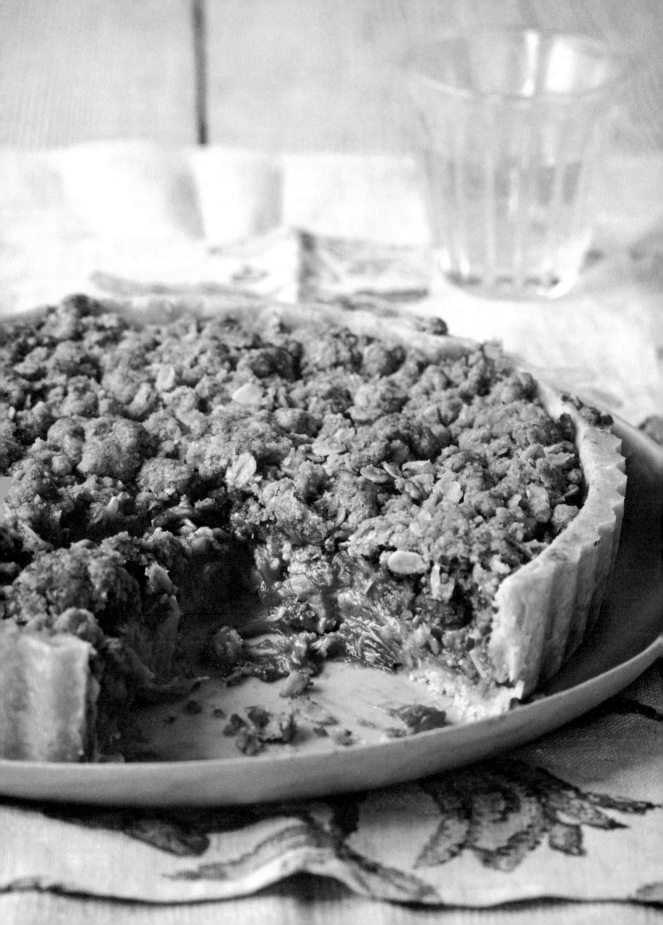

Drop Pancakes

Makes about 9 pancakes
—

125g/4½oz gluten-free
   self-raising flour
   (ideally Doves Farm)
A small pinch of sea salt
125ml/4½fl oz rice milk
1 heaped tsp egg replacer
   (ideally Orgran)
   whisked with 2 tbsp
   water
3 tsp Pure Sunflower
   Spread (dairy-free
   margarine)

For Apple and Cinnamon
1 peeled and grated
   eating apple
1 tsp ground cinnamon
Agave syrup, for drizzling

For Chocolate Chip
30g/1¼oz dairy-free
   dark chocolate, roughly
   chopped, or chocolate nibs
Pure Sunflower
   Spread (dairy-free
   margarine), to serve

For Lemon and Sugar
Grated zest and juice
   of 1 lemon
Caster sugar, for sprinkling

These pancakes are so simple to make and there are so many different ways of serving them. Here I've included instructions for making spicy Apple and Cinnamon, indulgent Chocolate Chip and classic Lemon and Sugar. The plain pancakes would also taste delicious served with a little stewed rhubarb (see page 58) for a seasonal touch.

Sift the flour and salt into a large bowl, add the rice milk and egg replacer mixture and whisk until you have a smooth, fluffy batter. Add any extra ingredients (if using) to the batter – grated apple and cinnamon (for Apple and Cinnamon), chocolate nibs (for Chocolate Chip) or lemon zest (for Lemon and Sugar) – and stir into the mixture until combined.

Add a teaspoon of the margarine to a large frying pan and melt over a medium heat. It is best to cook the pancakes in batches, three at a time, replenishing the margarine each time you cook a new batch and keeping the previously cooked pancakes warming in the oven, covered with foil or a clean tea towel. Carefully spoon in the batter – using roughly 1 rounded tablespoon of batter for each pancake – and use the back of the spoon to shape each pancake into a round.

Fry for 2–3 minutes or until golden underneath and then flip over to cook the other side for a further couple of minutes or until golden. Once the pancakes are cooked and slightly risen, transfer to individual plates. To serve, either drizzle with agave syrup (for Apple and Cinnamon) or add a knob of margarine to each pancake (for Chocolate Chip) or lemon juice and sugar (for Lemon and Sugar).

Flapjacks

Makes 9 squares
One variation
contains nuts

—

60g/2oz Pure Sunflower
   Spread (dairy-free
   margarine)
50g/1¾oz soft light
   brown sugar
100g/3½oz golden syrup
110g/4oz porridge oats
A small pinch of sea salt

For Almond
100g/3½oz flaked almonds

For Apple and Cinnamon
75g/3oz baked apples
   pieces (see page 205)

For Cranberry and Spice
75g/3oz dried cranberries
½ tsp mixed spice

For Sultana and Apricot
75g/3oz mixed sultanas
   and chopped dried
   apricots

*You will need a 20cm/8in
square baking tin for this
recipe*

As someone who suffers from multiple food intolerances, I think it's really useful to have a few recipes for snacks that you can take out and about with you. Flapjacks (or indeed, my Apple and Cinnamon Granola Bars – see page 205) are just the thing to pop in your bag or a side pocket of the car, ready to provide a quick boost of energy when needed. They are particularly versatile as you can vary the basic recipe in so many different ways. From Almond, Apple and Cinnamon, Cranberry and Spice to Sultana and Apricot, there will always be one to suit your mood. If stored in an airtight container, they will keep for up to a week – although I'll be surprised if they last that long!

Preheat the oven to 180°C/350°F/gas mark 4, then lightly grease and line the base of the baking tin with baking parchment.

Gently melt the margarine, sugar and golden syrup together in a large saucepan over a low heat, stirring occasionally, until you have a smooth liquid.

Add the oats and salt to the pan, along with the ingredients for one of the variations (if using), and stir until combined, then spread the flapjack mixture into the baking tin, levelling the top of the mixture with the back of the spoon.

Bake in the oven for 15 minutes or until the flapjacks are golden in colour but still slightly gooey in texture. Remove from the oven, cut into squares and then leave in the tin to cool completely. Once cooled, carefully lift the flapjacks (resting on the baking parchment) out of the tin and then use a sharp knife to re-cut the flapjack into squares before serving or storing in an airtight container.

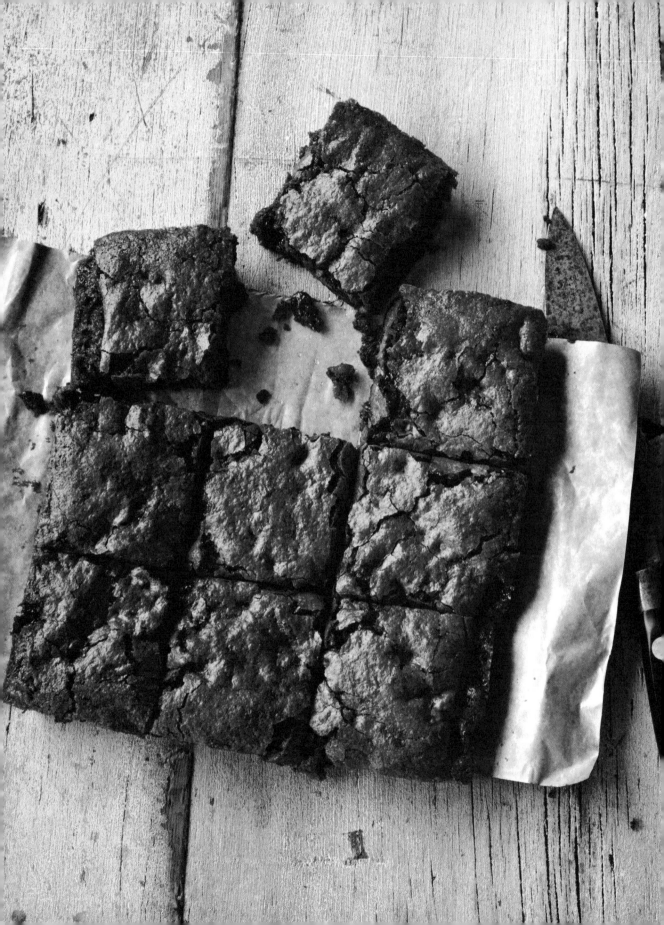

Chocolate Nut Brownies

Makes 12 brownies
Contains nuts

—

100g/3½oz Pure
Sunflower Spread
(dairy-free margarine),
plus extra for greasing
4 tbsp ground flaxseeds
¼ tsp baking powder
6 tbsp rice milk
50g/1¾oz dairy-free
dark chocolate
25g/1oz shelled walnuts
25g/1oz shelled pecan
nuts
175g/6oz soft light
brown sugar
½ tsp vanilla extract
100g/3½oz gluten-free
self-raising flour
(ideally Doves Farm)
A small pinch of sea salt

*You will need an 18cm/7in
square non-stick brownie
tin for this recipe*

The richness of the dark chocolate in these brownies is offset by the chopped nuts, the crisp chocolaty layer on top of each giving way to a divinely sticky centre. Brownies are meant to be intense, tender and gooey, so using flaxseeds to replace the egg in this recipe is ideal. Ground flaxseeds, although great as a binder, aren't always my first choice in baking as they can create a gummy centre. In this particular case, however, they only add to the texture of the cakes, heightening their intensity and sheer moreishness.

Preheat the oven to 180°C/350°F/gas mark 4, then lightly grease the brownie tin and line the base with baking parchment.

Whisk together the ground flaxseeds, baking powder and rice milk until blended, then set aside for a few minutes. The flax will swell up and absorb the rice milk so that you are left with a thick paste rather than a liquid.

Place a heatproof bowl over a saucepan containing 2.5cm/1in of simmering water, break up the chocolate and place it in the bowl with the margarine. Melt gently, stirring occasionally, until smooth and combined, then remove from the heat and set aside to cool down a little.

Meanwhile, roughly chop the nuts. Once the chocolate is cool enough to touch, stir in the sugar, flaxseed mixture and vanilla extract until fully amalgamated. Transfer to a large bowl and then sift in the flour, folding it in with the chopped nuts and a very small pinch of salt (which will do wonders for the intensity of the chocolate).

Pour the mixture into the prepared tin, spreading it out evenly and levelling the top with the back of a spoon, then bake in the oven for 25–30 minutes or until the top has crisped up slightly but the cake is still gooey in the middle. (You can use a skewer or cocktail stick to test this.) Leave to cool in the tin completely before cutting into squares and serving.

Jam Tarts

Makes 18–20 tartlets

—

1 quantity of sweet
  Shortcrust Pastry
  (see page 223)

For the filling
A jar of your favourite jam
  such as raspberry,
  strawberry, apricot
  or blackcurrant

*You will need a
6cm/2½in diameter
cookie cutter and two
12-hole tart tins for
this recipe*

*There's no substitute for a jam tart – or not for the finished article.
I love the hit of vibrant, syrupy fruit when you bite into one, followed
by the short, buttery pastry. These tarts are popular with children (and
adults!) of all ages and so are perfect for afternoon teas, picnics or parties.
Choose whatever flavour jam, or jams, you like for the filling. My only
recommendation would be the two-spoonful trick – it makes for the
most wonderfully, well, jammy tarts!*

Preheat the oven to 180°C/350°F/gas mark 4.

Roll out the pastry following the instructions given in the Shortcrust
Pastry recipe on page 223 and use the cookie cutter to cut out as many
little tarts as you can, kneading and re-rolling the pastry as necessary.
Carefully fit each circle into the holes of the tart tins, pressing the pastry
into the curves and using extra pastry to fill any cracks that may appear.

Place one teaspoonful of jam in each tart, then bake in the oven for
13–15 minutes or until the pastry is cooked and the jam is bubbling.
Remove the tin from the oven and immediately add another
teaspoonful of jam to each tart, carefully mixing this with the cooked
jam. Transfer the finished tarts to a wire rack and tuck in when they're
cool enough to eat!

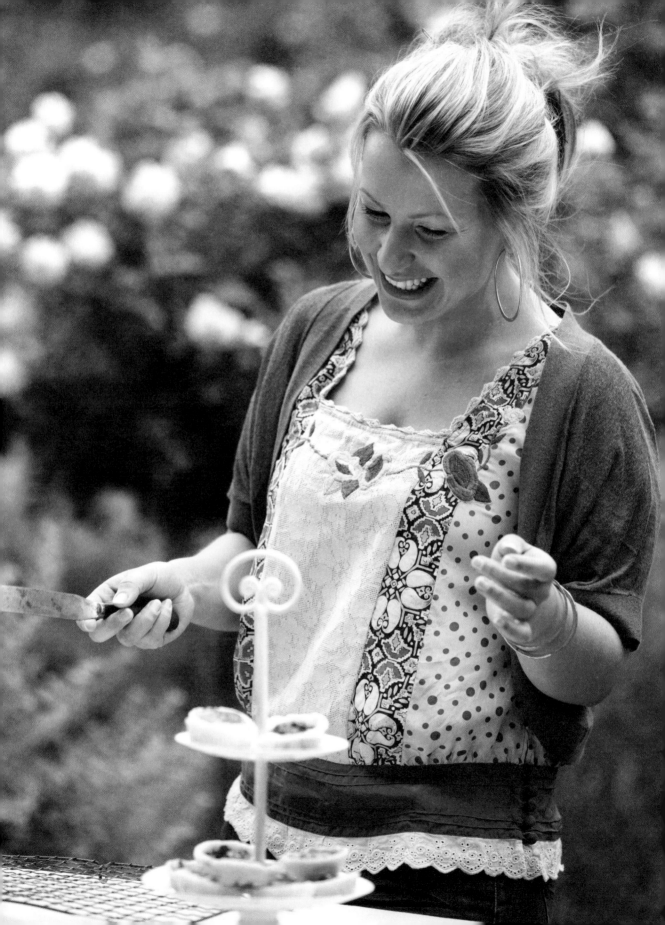

Chocolate Shortbread with Vanilla Ice Cream

Serves 4–6

—

For the ice cream
350ml/12fl oz almond
  or oat milk
250ml/9fl oz oat cream
50g/1¾oz golden caster
  sugar
1 tsp vanilla extract
Seeds from 1 vanilla pod

For the shortbread
100g/3½oz Pure
  Sunflower Spread
  (dairy-free margarine)
50g/1¾oz golden caster
  sugar
50g/1¾oz gluten-free
  plain flour (ideally
  Doves Farm)
25g/1oz cocoa powder
A small pinch of sea salt

*You will need cookie cutters
and an ice-cream maker
(minimum capacity of
1 litre/1¾ pints) for this
recipe if not making the
ice cream by hand*

*These shortbread biscuits have an intense cocoa flavour and a light,
delicate texture. They would be perfect for afternoon tea, but I like to serve
them as a pudding, crumbled over a scoop or two of this velvety vanilla ice
cream. You can make them together, or separately, of course – the choice is
yours. But, combined, they make the most indulgent treat.*

First make the shortbread. Cream together the margarine and sugar in
a large bowl. Sift in the flour, cocoa powder and salt and beat together
before covering the bowl and chilling in the fridge for 1 hour.

Preheat the oven to 180°C/350°F/gas mark 4 and line a baking sheet
with baking parchment.

Using a spatula or spoon, spread the shortbread mixture out on the
prepared baking sheet into an oblong shape, approximately 20 x 28cm/
8 x 11in in size and 5mm/¼in thick, and gently level the top. Bake in
the oven for 10 minutes or until slightly crispy at the edges. Pressing
the mixture lightly on top should leave an impression; once cooled,
the shortbread will firm up and become very 'short' and crumbly.

Remove from the oven and allow to cool for a few minutes. Then,
using a cookie cutter of your choice, cut out as many shortbread
biscuits as you can from the mixture and carefully transfer to a wire
rack to allow them to cool completely.

Meanwhile, prepare the ice cream. Place the almond or oat milk in
a large saucepan with the oat cream, sugar, vanilla extract and seeds
and set over a medium heat, whisking constantly, until the sugar has
completely dissolved. Set the mixture aside to cool down. Once cool,
refrigerate for 10 minutes before pouring into the ice-cream maker
and churning for 20–30 minutes. (Keep an eye on the ice cream while
it is churning to catch it when it has become creamy and smooth in
consistency, just past being 'soft set'.)

Alternatively, you can make the ice cream by hand – although I cannot
guarantee that it will be as smooth. Pour the cooled mixture into a
freezer-proof container or plastic tub and freeze for 1 hour or until
solid. Remove from the freezer, cut into rough chunks and, using a
hand-held blender or a food processor, blitz until smooth. Place the ice
cream in the fridge and leave for a further hour before blitzing again.

Once the ice cream is made (whether in the ice-cream maker or by
hand), it can be served immediately for soft-set ice cream or, alternatively,
poured into a freezer-proof container, covered with cling film and
frozen for at least 3 hours before serving.

Apricot Spice Sticky Squares

Makes 12 squares
Contains nuts

—

175g/6oz Pure Sunflower
  Spread (dairy-free
  margarine), plus
  extra for greasing
175g/6oz soft light
  brown sugar
175g/6oz soft dried
  apricots
2 tsp mixed spice
3 heaped tsp egg replacer
  (ideally Orgran)
  whisked with 6 tbsp
  water
1 tbsp rice milk
110g/4oz gluten-free
  plain flour (ideally
  Doves Farm)
¾ tsp bicarbonate
  of soda
½ tsp xanthan gum
225g/8oz ground
  almonds
3 tbsp agave syrup,
  to glaze

You will need a 20cm/
8in square cake tin
for this recipe

These cake squares have a wonderfully mellow, spicy undertone. The sticky part is down to the combination of the sugary apricot mixture and the ground almonds that make up the body of the cake. The agave syrup glaze adds a gloss and extra gooeyness to the whole affair. These will last for up to four days in an airtight tin, and actually improve in texture the day after baking.

Place the margarine, sugar and apricots in a saucepan (preferably non-stick) and add 3 tablespoons of water. Melt the mixture together, stirring occasionally, and then bring to the boil, boiling the mixture for exactly 5 minutes. Take the pan off the heat and set aside to cool down until you can dip your finger in without burning yourself. The mixture will be very hot, so do wait for at least 30 minutes before testing the temperature with your finger.

Preheat the oven to 150°C/300°F/gas mark 2, then lightly grease the cake tin and line the base and sides with baking parchment.

Once the apricot mixture has cooled, transfer to a large bowl. Beat in the mixed spice and then, while still beating, add the egg replacer mixture and rice milk. Sift in the flour, bicarbonate of soda and xanthan gum and then fold in the ground almonds, mixing together until fully combined.

Tip the cake mixture into the prepared tin, level the top and bake in the oven for 1 hour or until a skewer or cocktail stick inserted into the centre of the cake comes out clean. Carefully lift the cake out of the tin and allow to cool completely on a wire rack. Once cool, pour over the agave syrup and spread evenly with a spatula. Leave to set for 30 minutes and then cut into squares to serve.

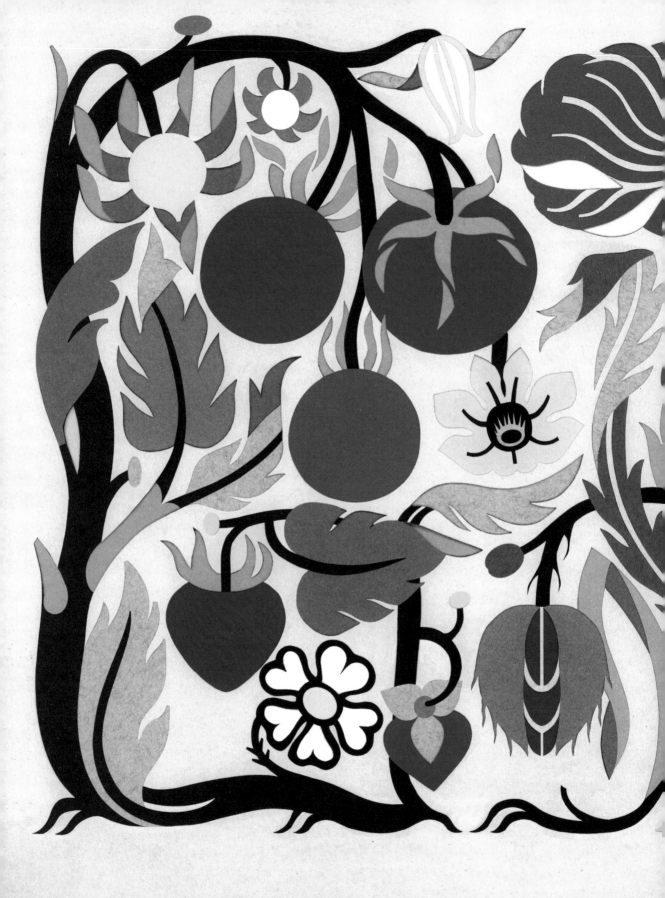

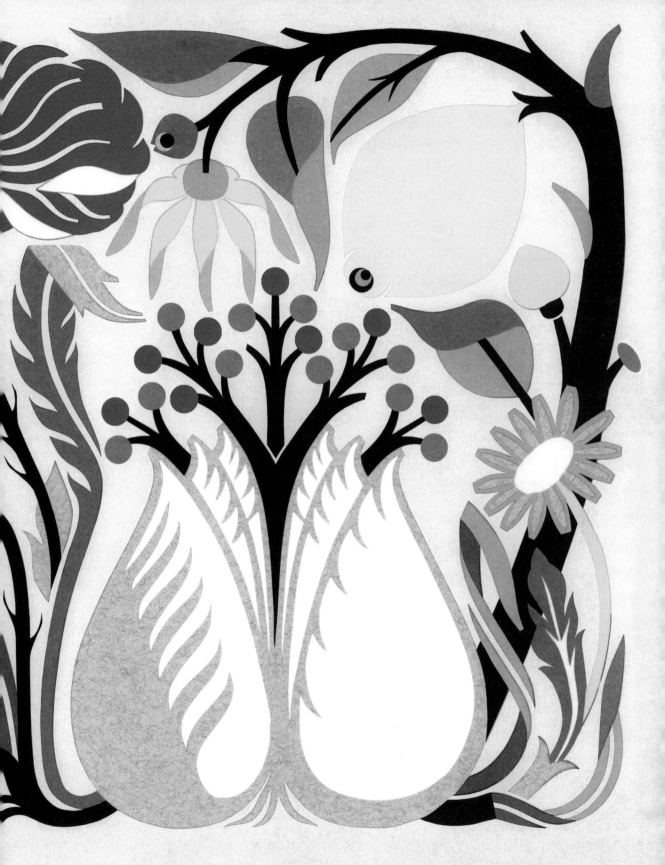

Summer

Sun-filled days call for colourful and effortless dishes, vibrant in appearance and varied in texture. This is the time for crunchy salads, sizzling meats, aromatic fresh herbs and light, fruity puddings. Dishes such as Seared Steaks with Roasted Pepper and Almond Sauce and Summer Tomato and Pesto Tart (see pages 94 and 96) are ideal for weekend barbecues or al fresco eating. The Roasted Aubergine and Quinoa Salad (see page 101) makes good use of the abundance of seasonal vegetables on offer, while creamy Chocolate Ice Cream (see page 113) provides the perfect finish for a light summer meal.

Chorizo, Chickpea and Spinach Salad

Serves 4

—

225g/8oz cooking chorizo
2 courgettes
A small bunch of
curly-leaf parsley
A small bunch of chives
12 cherry tomatoes
1 x 400g tin of chickpeas,
drained and rinsed
150g/5oz baby-leaf
spinach
1 tbsp extra-virgin
olive oil
Sea salt and freshly
ground black pepper

This is a gloriously colourful and tasty summer salad. The classic combination of chickpeas and chorizo is given added flavour with tender young spinach and sweet, juicy cherry tomatoes. It makes a wonderful starter or light lunch when served with my homemade Flatbreads (see page 221). A quick word about chorizo: this authentic Spanish sausage can be found in most delis and big supermarkets. Be sure to check the ingredients carefully; they can occasionally contain dairy produce or wheat, but there should always be at least one brand that is allergen-free.

Prepare the chorizo by slicing it in half lengthways and then cut into half-moons approximately 1cm/½in thick. Trim the courgettes and cut them to the same proportions, then roughly chop the herbs and slice the cherry tomatoes into a mixture of halves and quarters.

Heat a large, heavy-based frying pan over a medium heat until hot. Add the chorizo and courgettes and fry for about 10 minutes, stirring frequently, until the chorizo releases its paprika oil and starts to become crisp on the outside. Remove from the heat and set aside to cool.

In a large bowl, combine the chickpeas, spinach, chopped herbs and tomatoes, season with salt and pepper and mix together. Add the fried courgettes and chorizo, drizzle over the olive oil, toss together thoroughly and serve.

Slow-roasted Tomatoes

Serves 4

—

6 plum or vine-ripened
 tomatoes
4 tbsp olive oil
4 tbsp soft light brown
 sugar
Extra-virgin olive oil,
 for drizzling
Sea salt and freshly
 ground black pepper

These tomatoes have a lovely depth of flavour – sweet, rich and tangy and a real pleasure to eat. Years ago, I spent six months in Italy and discovered the delights of antipasti, of which roasted tomatoes are a staple ingredient. With this recipe, I hope to have recreated something approaching that Italian dish. You could serve the tomatoes as part of your own platter of antipasti, with some salami, bresaola and a salad of rocket, avocado and preserved artichoke hearts. At the very least, they are a wonderful standby for adding to sauces and stirring into pasta, rice and other grains, such as my Tomato, Basil and Pine Nut Quinoa (see page 104). For a slightly more complex flavour, you could add a very fine sliver of garlic and a light sprinkling of dried oregano to each tomato half before baking in the oven.

Preheat the oven to 110°C/225°F/gas mark ¼.

Cut the tomatoes in half lengthways and, using a teaspoon, carefully scoop out the seeds and pith, being sure not to tear through the tomato skin.

Place each tomato half, skin side down, on a baking tray. Carefully pour 1 teaspoon each of olive oil and sugar into each tomato half, then sprinkle liberally with salt and pepper.

Bake in the oven for 1½–2 hours or until the tomatoes are softened and roasted but not overly browned or caramelised. Remove from the oven, set aside and leave to cool completely – this will take a couple of hours. Once cool, place in an airtight container and drizzle liberally with extra-virgin olive oil. If refrigerated, these will keep for up to two weeks.

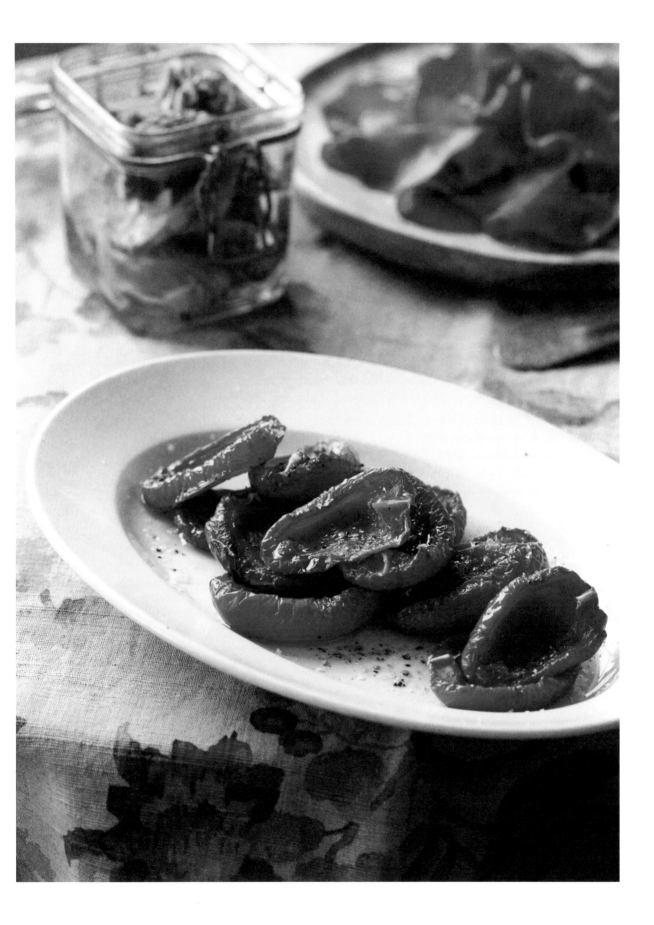

Crayfish, Mango and Avocado Salad

Serves 4

—

2 ripe Hass avocados
1 ripe mango
A small bunch of chives
A small bunch of coriander
1 small red chilli
400g/14oz cooked and
    peeled crayfish tails
Juice of ½ lemon
4 Little Gem lettuces
2 tbsp extra-virgin olive oil
Sea salt and freshly
    ground black pepper

This simple salad makes a delicious starter for four people or serves two as a light lunch; it is delicate and refreshing with a glow of chilli – perfect for a summer's day and al fresco eating. If you would like to make it for more, just double the quantities accordingly. I like to use Hass avocados as they have a distinctive creamy texture that contrasts with the bite of the Gem lettuce and the tender flesh of the mango and crayfish.

Slice each avocado in half, remove the stone and, using a spoon, scoop out the flesh. Peel the mango, removing the stone, then cut the avocado and mango flesh into 1cm/½in cubes. Finely chop the chives and coriander, then deseed the chilli and slice into fine half-rings. Rinse the crayfish tails with cold water and pat dry with kitchen paper.

In a large bowl, combine the crayfish tails with the chopped avocado, mango and herbs. Squeeze over the lemon juice and season with salt and pepper. Cover and chill in the fridge for 30–60 minutes to allow the flavours to infuse.

When ready to serve, break up the lettuces into leaves, divide between plates and drizzle with the olive oil. Remove the crayfish mixture from the fridge and carefully pile onto the lettuce leaves, scatter over the chilli and serve immediately.

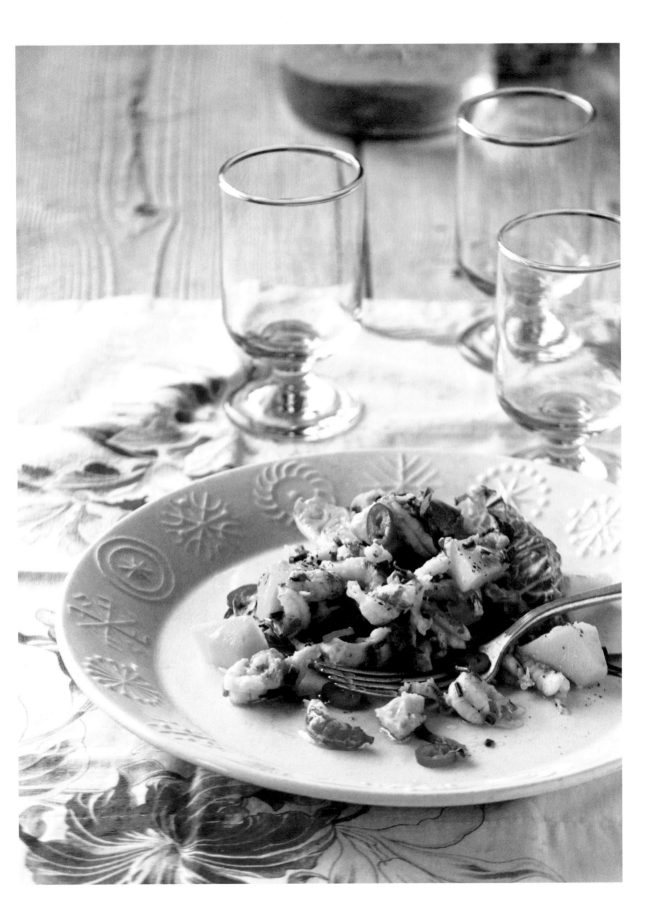

Prawn and Pineapple Rice Salad

Serves 4
Contains nuts
—
175g/6oz Carmague
   red rice
500ml/18fl oz vegetable
   stock
50g/1¾oz sultanas
25g/1oz flaked almonds
200g/7oz cooked and
   peeled prawns
225g/8oz fresh pineapple
2 spring onions
A bunch of coriander
1 tbsp toasted sesame oil
½ tsp turmeric
Sea salt and freshly ground
   black pepper

This might seem like an odd combination of flavours but it really works, the sweetness of the pineapple, sultanas and prawns complemented by the nutty bite of the almonds and red rice and the dusky undertone of the turmeric. This is a lovely salad to eat in the summertime – bright and fragrant, it's all the better for being served on a bed of fresh green leaves. Everyone has their own way of cooking rice, but I find the absorption method the most reliable. A simple way of ensuring you always get it right is to use double the volume of water or stock to rice. Hence if you're using one mugful of rice you would add two mugs of water or stock for perfectly cooked, fluffy grains.

Combine the rice and stock in a large saucepan, cover with a lid and bring to the boil. Once boiling, reduce the heat to low and simmer gently for 35 minutes or until the rice is tender and all the stock has been absorbed. When the rice is cooked, set aside and leave to cool completely.

Meanwhile, cover the sultanas with warm water and leave to soak for about 20 minutes or until soft, then drain and set aside.

In a heavy-based frying pan, dry-fry the flaked almonds over a medium heat for 3–4 minutes or until golden, shaking the pan regularly to ensure they don't burn. Once toasted, set aside to cool.

Rinse the prawns under cold water and pat dry with kitchen paper, then peel and chop the pineapple into 1cm/½in chunks, finely slice the spring onions into rounds and finely chop the coriander.

Once the rice has cooled, tip it into a large serving bowl. Drizzle over the sesame oil, season with salt, pepper and the turmeric and toss together before stirring in the pineapple, spring onions, sultanas, prawns and toasted almonds and scattering over the chopped coriander to serve.

Herb Pancakes with Smoked Salmon

Makes 12 pancakes

—

500g/1lb 2oz smoked
 salmon
Freshly ground black
 pepper
1 lemon, cut into
 8 wedges, to serve

For the pancakes
100g/3½oz gluten-free
 plain flour (ideally
 Doves Farm)
1 tsp baking powder
100ml/3½fl oz rice milk
2 heaped tsp egg replacer
 (ideally Orgran) whisked
 with 4 tbsp water
A small bunch of chives
A small bunch of coriander
A small bunch of curly-leaf
 parsley
1½ tbsp dairy-free
 margarine (ideally Pure
 Sunflower Spread)
Sea salt and freshly
 ground black pepper

Light and incredibly moreish, these are ideal as a starter, although they'd be great for a special brunch too, with a little fresh fruit (such as strawberries and blueberries or slices of apricot, peach or mango) and perhaps a glass of fizz alongside. The beauty of the dish lies in its simplicity and the enticingly fresh flavour of the chopped herbs. As you will have to make the pancakes in batches, I advise keeping them warm by wrapping them in foil or a clean tea towel and storing in the oven at a low temperature until you are ready to serve.

Sift the flour and baking powder into a large bowl. Season the flour well with salt and pepper and then gently whisk in the rice milk and egg replacer mixture. Finely chop the herbs and stir into the batter.

Add ½ tablespoon of the margarine to a large non-stick frying pan and melt over a medium heat. Carefully spoon in the batter – roughly 1 rounded tablespoon of batter for each pancake – using the back of the spoon to shape each pancake into a circle. Repeat this three more times so that you have four small pancakes in the pan, evenly spaced apart. Cook the pancakes for 1–2 minutes on each side or until they are golden and a little puffed up.

Remove from the pan and store (covered and kept in the oven, as recommended above) until ready to serve, then repeat the process until you have used up all the pancake batter, replenishing the margarine after each batch.

Once all the pancakes are prepared, lay three of them on each plate, drape over a quarter of the smoked salmon (carefully tearing it into strips before adding to the plates), add a grinding of pepper and a lemon wedge or two. Repeat the process with the remaining pancakes and salmon, and then serve.

Chicken and Noodle Salad with Spicy Peanut Dressing

Serves 4
Contains nuts

—

30g/1oz unsalted
  cashew nuts
2 skinless chicken breasts
½ tbsp toasted sesame oil
1 red pepper
¼ cucumber
300g/11oz rice noodles
Sea salt

*For the spicy peanut
dressing*
1 red chilli
A small bunch of coriander
2 tbsp smooth peanut
  butter
75ml/3fl oz coconut milk
1½ tsp soft light brown
  sugar
Juice of ½ lime
Sea salt and freshly
  ground black pepper

This salad is full of taste and texture, the chilli, coconut milk and peanut butter combining to create a creamy yet spicy dressing that offsets the crunchy red pepper and mild, tender chicken. You could serve it in four small portions as a starter or divide it into two larger servings for an intimate supper for two. If you don't fancy using chicken, then cooked prawns or salmon, lightly flaked, will work just as well.

Preheat the oven to 200°C/400°F/gas mark 6.

Scatter the cashew nuts on a baking tray and toast in the oven, turning them from time to time to make sure they don't burn, for 5–6 minutes or until golden brown, then remove, sprinkle with salt and set aside to cool.

Using a sharp knife and cutting to a depth of around 5mm/¼in, score each chicken breast diagonally three times and rub in the sesame oil. Place in a roasting tin and cook for 14 minutes, then remove from the oven and set aside to cool.

Meanwhile, make the dressing. Carefully deseed the chilli and finely chop until almost minced in texture, roughly chop the coriander and combine the two in a small bowl with the peanut butter, coconut milk, sugar and lime juice. Whip with a spoon until smooth and creamy and season with salt and pepper to taste.

Deseed the red pepper and cut lengthways into thin strips. Peel and cut the cucumber lengthways into strips about 5mm/¼in thick, then cut each strip into fine batons.

Once the chicken has cooled, cut widthways into fine slices. Cover the rice noodles in boiling water and leave for as long as instructed on the packet (usually around 10 minutes). Once soft and pliable, drain the noodles and place in a large serving bowl, combining them with the sliced chicken, red pepper and cucumber.

Add the dressing and mix thoroughly until evenly coated, then scatter over the toasted cashew nuts and toss again before serving.

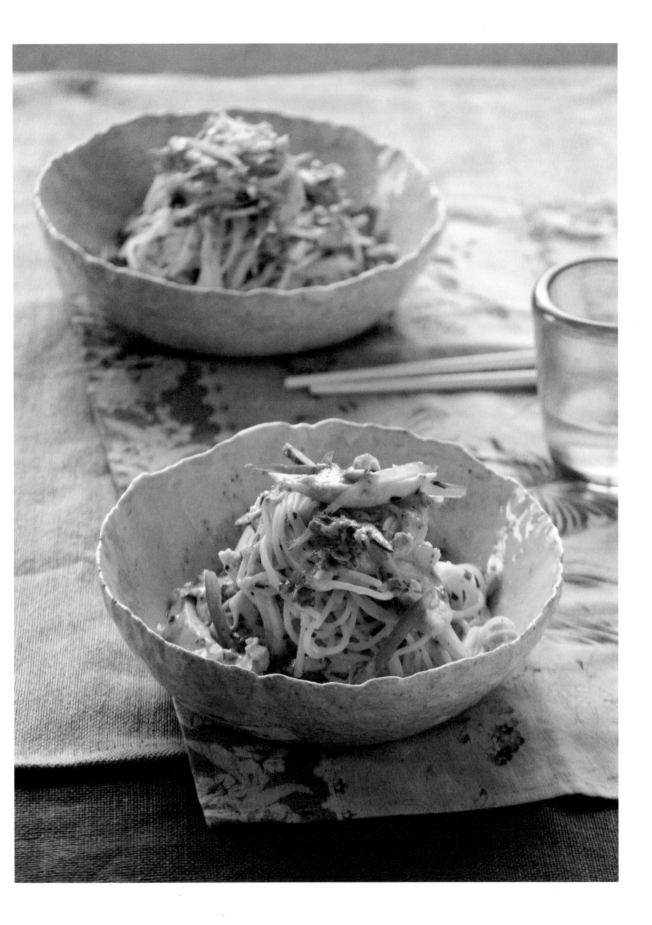

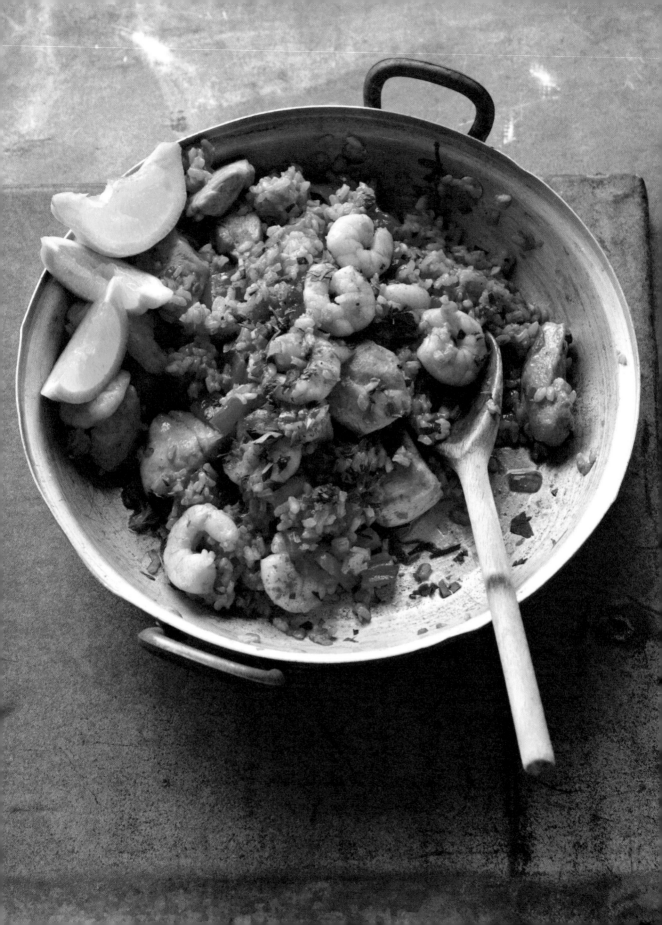

Chicken and Prawn Paella

Serves 4

—

2 skinless chicken breasts
1 large Spanish onion
3 cloves of garlic
2 red ramiro peppers
500ml/18fl oz chicken
  stock
1 tsp saffron threads
2 tbsp olive oil
1 tsp smoked paprika
1 tsp soft light brown sugar
175g/6oz paella rice
250g/9oz cooked and
  peeled tiger prawns
2 tsp lemon juice
Sea salt and freshly
  ground black pepper

*You will need a 30cm/12in
diameter paella pan or
heavy-based frying pan
with a lid for this recipe*

*I love the combination of tender chicken breasts and sweet tiger prawns
with saffron and smoked paprika. This is a fantastic dish to serve friends
and family for a relaxed supper – the kind of meal that you can cook while
chatting with loved ones, a glass of something cool and refreshing in one
hand. For maximum effect, cook and serve in a traditional paella pan or
spoon into a huge terracotta bowl and invite everyone to tuck in. I like it
served simply with a leafy green salad dressed with a little lemon juice
and olive oil. Pure heaven!*

Cut the chicken into 4cm/1½in chunks and set aside. Finely dice
the onion and crush the garlic, then deseed the peppers, cut in half
lengthways and slice widthways into strips about 5mm/¼in thick.

Pour the chicken stock into a saucepan, add the saffron and bring
to the boil. Once boiling, reduce the heat to its lowest setting so that
the stock remains hot, but without bubbling.

Pour the olive oil into the paella pan or frying pan and place over a
medium heat. Add the chicken and fry to seal the meat, turning it every
now and then, for approximately 5 minutes. Remove the chicken from
the pan and set aside, then lower the heat and gently fry the onions and
garlic for 5 minutes or until starting to soften.

Add the sliced peppers to the onion and fry gently over a low heat
until soft but not browned. Add the paprika and sugar, seasoning well
with salt and pepper, then return the chicken pieces to the pan and stir
all the ingredients together.

Next, add the rice to the chicken mixture and stir-fry over a medium
heat for 2 minutes or until the rice begins to turn glassy. Pour over the
hot stock, cover the pan with a lid and turn the heat down low. Leave to
cook for 40–45 minutes, occasionally giving the pan a gentle shake to
ensure the rice doesn't catch. If you think the stock is being absorbed
too quickly, simply add a little extra water to the pan.

Stir in the prawns, then drizzle over the lemon juice, cover again
with the lid and leave to cook for a further 5 minutes. The rice should
have absorbed all the stock at this point, tasting soft while still retaining
a little crunch. Remove the paella from the heat and serve.

Paprika Pepper Chicken with Avocado Salsa

Serves 4

—

1 red pepper

2 yellow peppers

2 red onions

4 cloves of garlic

A bunch of coriander

8 skinless and boneless
chicken thighs or 4
skinless chicken breasts

3 tbsp olive oil

2½ tsp smoked paprika

2½ tsp soft light brown
sugar

1 x 400g tin of chopped
tomatoes

Sea salt and freshly
ground black pepper

For the salsa

2 large firm tomatoes

1 red chilli

½ red onion

A small bunch of
coriander

1 ripe avocado

Juice of 1 lime

Sea salt and freshly
ground black pepper

This is a delightful meal for a balmy summer's evening, and perfect for using to fill some of my Corn Tortillas (see page 222). You can make the tortillas first and then keep them warm in the oven while you cook the chicken. The quantities for this recipe can easily be doubled, and if I'm serving it to lots of people I usually accompany it with white basmati rice and a cooling avocado salsa.

Deseed the peppers and cut lengthways into strips 5mm/¼in thick. Halve the onions and slice into thin half-moons. Crush the garlic and finely chop the coriander, then slice the chicken into strips approximately 1.5cm/⅝in thick.

Place the chicken in a large bowl and add the onions, peppers, garlic, olive oil, smoked paprika and sugar, mixing thoroughly to combine. Cover and leave somewhere cool to marinade for 1 hour.

Meanwhile, preheat the oven to 200°C/400°F/gas mark 6 and prepare the salsa.

First skin the tomatoes by placing them in a bowl, covering in boiling water and leaving for 1 minute. Drain and carefully peel away the tomato skins (they should slide off with ease), then slice in half, scoop out the seeds and finely dice the flesh.

Deseed the chilli and and finely chop this along with the onion and coriander. Halve the avocado, remove the stone and scoop out the flesh, then roughly chop and mix together with the tomatoes, chilli, coriander and lime juice. Season with salt and pepper, then cover with cling film and leave to chill in the fridge while you continue to cook.

Place the chicken and peppers in an ovenproof dish along with all the marinade and cook for 15 minutes, stirring occasionally, until softened and lightly browned.

Remove the chicken from the oven, pour over the chopped tomatoes, season with salt and pepper and stir together. Return to the oven and cook for a further 10–15 minutes, then remove from the oven, sprinkle with the chopped coriander and serve with the salsa on the side.

Sweet Chilli and Orange Chicken with Oriental Coleslaw

Serves 4
Contains nuts

—

2.5cm/1in piece
of root ginger
2 red chillies
2 spring onions
1 tbsp toasted sesame oil
2 tbsp lemon juice
Grated zest of 1 orange
and 2 tbsp orange juice
2 tbsp agave syrup or
soft light brown sugar
4 skinless chicken breasts
50g/1¾oz unsalted
cashew nuts
A bunch of coriander
Sea salt

For the coleslaw
1 Chinese cabbage
2 carrots
1 x 200g tin of sweetcorn,
drained and rinsed
1 tbsp toasted sesame oil
Sea salt and freshly
ground black pepper

This dish tastes like summertime in a bowl – I adore its zesty flavours and vivid colours. Perfect for a light lunch or supper, it is the kind of meal that leaves you feeling both satisfied and energised. The crunch of the cabbage, kick of the chilli and tender bite of the chicken combine with the zing of the orange and lemon to produce a well-balanced, vibrant dish. Chicken and coleslaw are perfectly suited, in my view, but you could cook the chicken on its own, allowing it to cool and then using it as a filling for sandwiches or baked potatoes; its citrus overtones work really well with creamy avocado.

Peel and finely grate the root ginger, then deseed the chillies and finely chop these and the spring onions. Place all these in a large bowl and mix with the sesame oil, lemon juice, orange zest and juice and agave syrup or brown sugar.

Using a sharp knife and cutting to a depth of around 1cm/½in, score each chicken breast diagonally 3–4 times. Place the chicken in the bowl with the marinade, turning to coat, and leave for 30 minutes to develop in flavour.

Meanwhile, preheat the oven to 200°C/400°F/gas mark 6.

Scatter the cashew nuts on a baking tray and toast in the oven, turning them from time to time to make sure they don't burn, for 5–6 minutes or until golden brown, then remove, sprinkle with salt and set aside to cool.

Next prepare the coleslaw. Finely slice the Chinese cabbage and cut the carrots into fine strips about 4cm/1½in long, then add all these to a large serving bowl. Tip in the sweetcorn, drizzle with the toasted sesame oil, season with salt and pepper and toss together.

Place the chicken breasts in a roasting tin, pour over the remaining marinade and cook in the oven for 15 minutes or until the juices run clear when the chicken is pierced with a skewer. Remove from the oven, cover in foil and allow to rest for 5 minutes. Once rested, cut the chicken breasts into slices 1cm/½in thick.

Divide the coleslaw between plates, adding pieces of the cooked chicken on top and pouring over the remaining juices. Finely chop the coriander and scatter this and the toasted cashew nuts over the chicken and coleslaw. Mix together gently and serve.

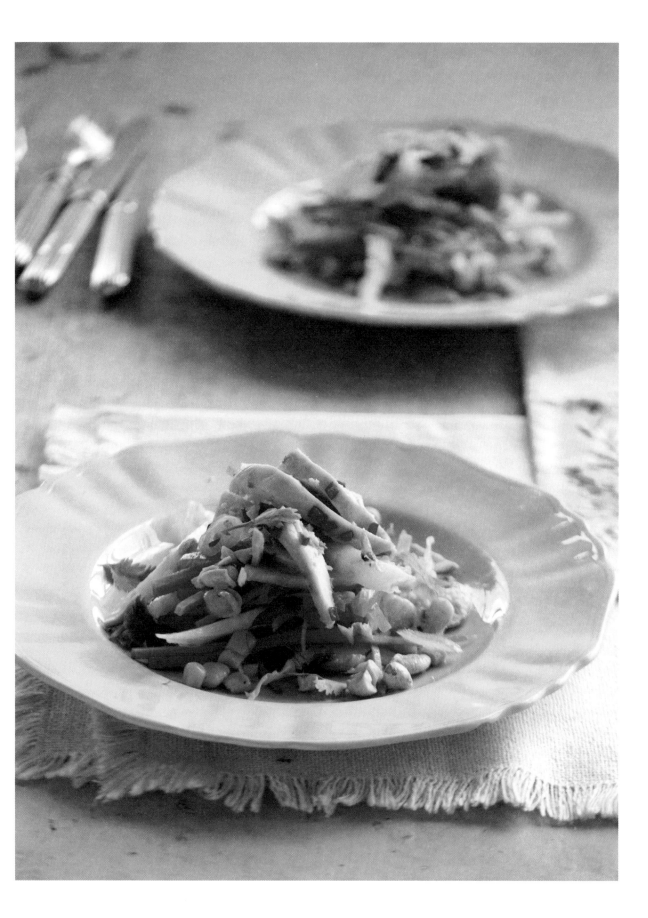

Pork Satay Skewers

Serves 4
Contains nuts
—

1kg/2lb 4oz pork fillet
2 large red peppers
4 spring onions

For the satay sauce
200ml/7fl oz coconut
    milk
2 tbsp crunchy peanut
    butter
5cm/2in piece of
    root ginger
2 cloves of garlic
1 red chilli
A bunch of coriander
1 tsp allergy-friendly
    stock powder
2 tsp soft light brown
    sugar
A good pinch of sea salt
2 tbsp warm water
1 tsp toasted sesame oil

*You will need eight bamboo
skewers, pre-soaked in
water for 30 minutes, or
eight metal skewers for
this recipe*

*This deliciously nutty, spiced dish is ideal for a summer's evening, its
bright flavour sweetened by the marrying of peanut and pork. I recommend
serving it with a bowl of steamed white basmati rice and a salad of ribboned
carrot and cucumber. The flavour of soy sauce is difficult to replicate, but
I find that by using a blend of toasted sesame oil, seasoning and stock
powder you can recreate the 'umami' flavour that is so fundamental
to this type of cooking.*

First make the satay sauce. Gently heat the coconut milk in a small
saucepan. Add the peanut butter and stir continuously over a low heat
until it has dissolved and you are left with a thick sauce. Take off the
heat and set aside.

Peel the ginger and finely grate both this and the garlic. Finely
chop the chilli, retaining the seeds, and coriander and add to a bowl
with the ginger and garlic. Add the stock powder, sugar, salt, warm
water and sesame oil and then mix together. Pour over the peanut
and coconut milk and stir together before dividing the sauce between
two separate bowls.

Trim any excess fat from the pork fillet and cut into 2.5cm/1in
chunks. Add the pork to one bowl of the satay sauce, mix thoroughly,
cover and leave to marinate for 30 minutes to 3 hours (don't refrigerate
as this tends to make the coconut milk solidify). Set aside the remaining
sauce, also covered, for later.

While the pork is marinating, deseed the pepper and cut into 2.5cm/
1in pieces. Finely chop the spring onion into rounds and set aside.

When you are ready to cook, preheat the grill to medium–high.

Thread the marinated pork onto the skewers, alternating every now
and then with the chunks of red pepper. Place under the grill and cook
for 10–15 minutes, turning occasionally, until the pork is cooked and
tender. Remove from the grill, place on a serving platter, sprinkle over
the spring onions and serve with a bowl of white basmati rice and the
remaining satay sauce to dip the pork into.

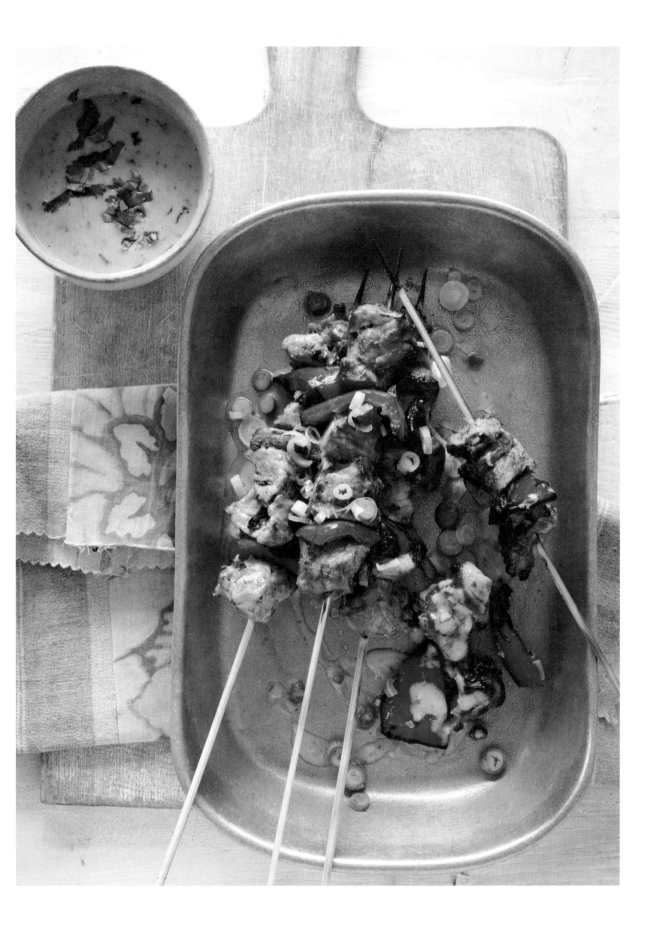

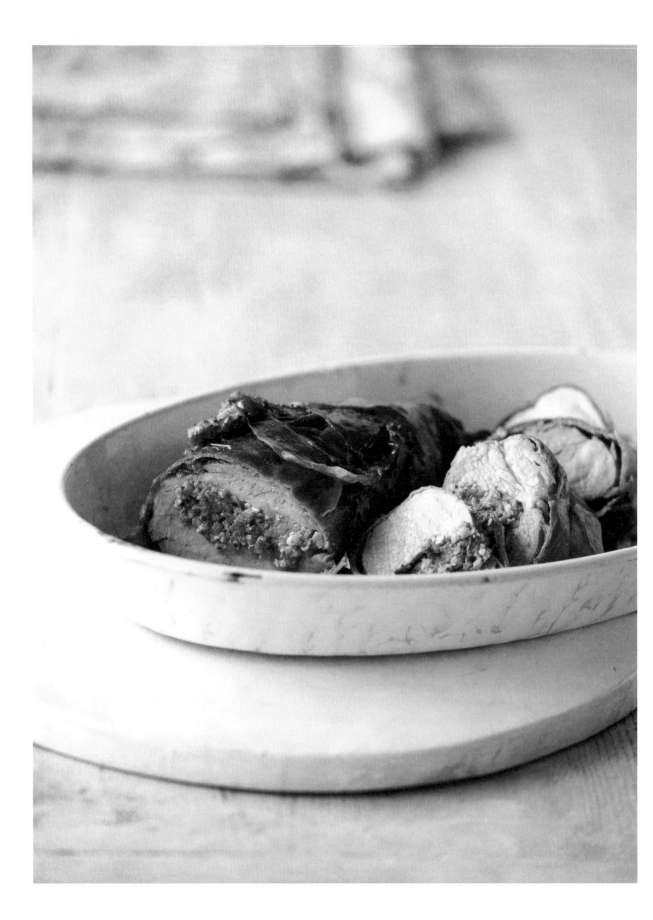

Pork Tenderloin filled with Tomato Pesto

Serves 4
Contains nuts
—
Olive oil, for drizzling
2 x 400g/14oz pork
  tenderloin fillets
12 slices of Parma ham

For the pesto
100g/3½oz pine nuts
100g/3½oz sun-blushed
  tomatoes
Leaves from a large
  bunch of basil
Leaves from 6 sprigs
  of thyme
3 tbsp extra-virgin
  olive oil
Sea salt and freshly
  ground black pepper

This pesto is a heavenly blend of sweet, sun-blushed tomatoes, toasted pine nuts and fragrant basil and thyme. It is used to fill the pork tenderloin fillets, which are then wrapped in Parma ham, forming a salty, crisp outer layer that preserves the succulence and flavour of the meat. It is delicious served with steamed or roasted new potatoes and drizzled with olive oil.

Preheat the oven to 190°C/375°F/gas mark 5 and lightly drizzle a baking tray with olive oil.

Next make the pesto. Scatter the pine nuts over another baking tray and toast in the oven, turning them from time to time to make sure they don't burn, for 5–6 minutes or until golden brown, then remove from the oven and set aside to cool.

Roughly chop the sun-blushed tomatoes and place in a food processor with the basil and thyme leaves, toasted pine nuts and a good pinch of salt. Pour in the olive oil and briefly blitz to a coarse pesto. Alternatively, pound the ingredients together using a pestle and mortar. (Depending on the size of your mortar, you may have to do this in two batches.) Taste the pesto, adding a little extra salt or some pepper if you think it needs it, cover with cling film and store in the fridge until you are ready to use it.

Place the pork tenderloin fillets on a chopping board and, using a small sharp knife, trim any excess fat from around the meat. Next, place the point of your knife in the centre of the tenderloin and slice along its length, cutting about 1cm/½in deep, but not all the way through, so that you can carefully open out the meat and fill the centre of it. Repeat with the second tenderloin.

Carefully spoon the pesto along the centre of each opened-out fillet, spreading the pesto along its length, and then roll or fold the pork back together so that the pesto is sandwiched in the centre of the meat.

Lay out six slices of the Parma ham horizontally on your chopping board, ensuring each edge overlaps slightly, and then carefully lay one of the pork fillets vertically on top. Wrap the ham around the tenderloin, tucking in the edges so that it forms a tight package. Repeat with the second tenderloin, wrapping it in the remaining slices of Parma ham.

Place the meat on the baking tray drizzled with olive oil, cover with foil and bake in the oven for 10 minutes. Remove the foil and return the tenderloins to the oven for a further 15–20 minutes or until the ham is crisp and the pork cooked through, the juices running clear when the meat is pierced with a skewer. Re-cover the meat with the foil and leave to rest for 10 minutes before cutting into slices and serving.

Butterflied Leg of Lamb with Olive and Mint Tapenade

Serves 4–6
Contains nuts

—

2kg/4½lb butterflied leg of lamb (ask your butcher to prepare this for you)
6 cloves of garlic
2 tbsp olive oil
Sea salt and freshly ground black pepper

For the tapenade
100g/3½oz pine nuts
A large bunch of mint
50g/1¾oz pitted black olives
3 tbsp extra-virgin olive oil
Freshly ground black pepper

This variation on the traditional theme of lamb and mint is perfect for summer eating. Carving through the tender lamb reveals piquant stubs of roasted garlic and a layer of garden-fresh tapenade, imbuing the meat with an intense flavour, evocative of the Mediterranean. I quite often serve it with a large bowl of my Ratatouille and Potatoes with Parsley, Capers and Lemon (see pages 99 and 104) – the flavours go really well together. But it's equally delicious served cold, with a baked potato and a green salad on the side.

Preheat the oven to 200°C/400°F/gas mark 6.

First make the tapenade. Scatter the pine nuts over a baking tray and toast in the oven, turning them from time to time to make sure they don't burn, for 5–6 minutes or golden brown, then remove from the oven and set aside to cool. Reduce the oven temperature to 180°C/350°F/gas mark 4.

Place the toasted pine nuts in a food processor with the mint, olives and olive oil, season with a little pepper, and blitz until you have a coarse tapenade.

Lay out the lamb – fat side down – on a chopping board and spread the tapenade all over the top of the meat. Carefully roll up the lamb, folding in the edges to enclose the filling, and secure with string or butcher's twine so that you have an oval roll of meat.

Halve each garlic clove lengthways, then place the lamb in a large roasting tin and, using a small sharp knife, make twelve 1cm/½in incisions all over the meat. Insert a shard of garlic into each incision, then drizzle over the olive oil. Season well with salt and pepper and roast in the oven for 1½–2 hours (1½ hours for lamb that is still slightly pink in the middle) or until the meat is cooked through and tender. Remove the lamb from the oven, cover with foil and leave to rest for 20 minutes before carving.

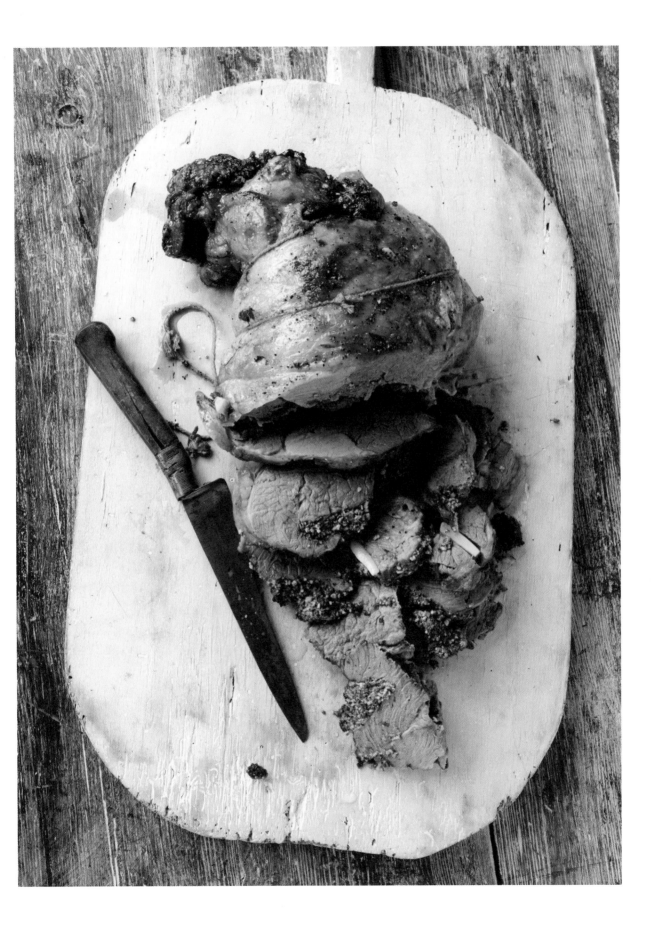

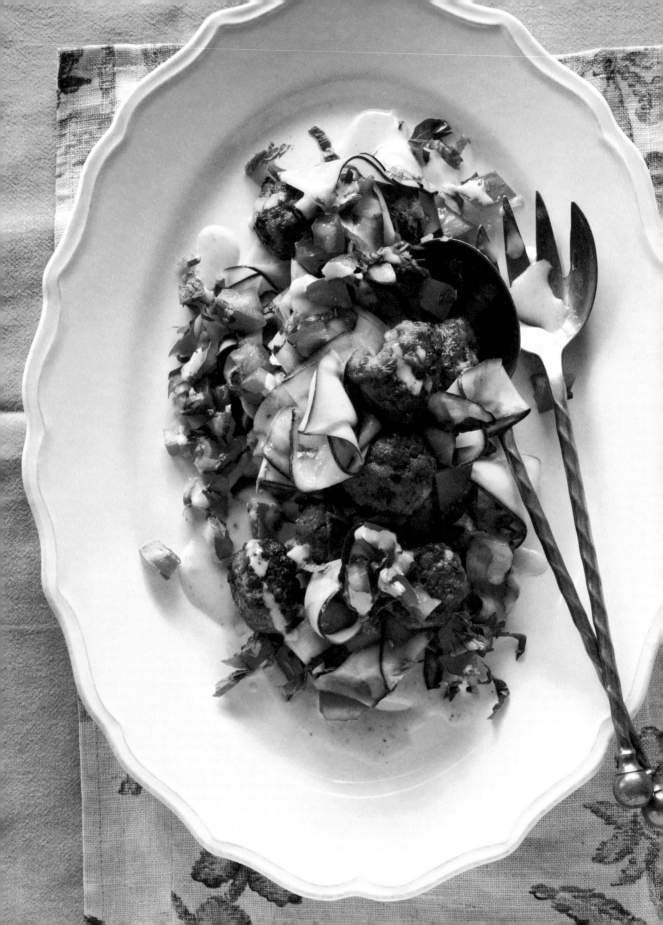

Greek Meatballs with Griddled Courgette and Tomato Salad and Tahini Dressing

Serves 4

—

For the meatballs

1 red onion
A small bunch of mint
2 tbsp olive oil
250g/9oz lean minced
    lamb
250g/9oz lean minced
    pork
½ tsp cumin
Sea salt and freshly
    ground black pepper

For the salad

6 courgettes
4 large vine-ripened
    tomatoes
A small bunch of
    flat-leaf parsley
A small bunch of mint
1 tbsp olive oil
Juice of ¼ lemon
Sea salt and freshly
    ground black pepper

For the dressing

2 tbsp tahini paste
½ clove of garlic
1 tbsp lemon juice
1 tsp agave syrup
¼ tsp ground cumin
Sea salt and freshly
    ground black pepper

There is really only one way to eat this dish (which I highly recommend that you do) and that is as a simple platter accompanied with Flatbreads (see page 221), houmous and a scattering of kalamata olives. This recipe makes approximately 40 meatballs; I know that ten meatballs each may sound like far too many, but trust me – they are very small and very moreish; you will be grateful for the excess!

Begin by preparing the dressing. Add the tahini paste to a small bowl and stir in 2–3 tablespoons of water, bit by bit, until you have a smooth, thin paste. Crush the garlic and mix into the paste with the lemon juice, agave syrup and cumin, then season with salt and pepper to taste – you can add more lemon juice or agave syrup if you feel it needs it.

To start preparing the meatballs, dice the onion very finely and finely chop the mint. Add 1 tablespoon of the olive oil to a frying pan and sauté the onion gently over a medium heat for 5–6 minutes or until completely tender and translucent but not browned. Season with salt and pepper and set aside to cool slightly.

Next top and tail the courgettes for the salad and, using a wide vegetable peeler, peel into fine ribbons, discarding the outer peelings. Finely chop the tomatoes, parsley and mint. Place the courgettes in a bowl with the olive oil, season well with salt and pepper and mix until thoroughly coated. Heat a griddle pan or heavy-based frying pan until very hot and fry the courgette ribbons (in batches) for 3–4 minutes or until slightly softened and charred. Remove from the pan, drizzle with the lemon juice and set aside.

Preheat the oven to 190°C/375°F/gas mark 5.

Place the minced lamb and pork in a large bowl and combine with the cumin, chopped mint and cooked onion, season well with salt and pepper and mix together with your hands. Pinch off a small amount of the mixture and, rolling it between the palms of your hands, shape into a ball approximately 2.5cm/1in in diameter. Repeat with the rest of the mixture, then place the meatballs in a large roasting tin, spaced evenly apart, and drizzle with the remaining olive oil. Cook in the oven for 12–14 minutes, turning occasionally, until cooked through and nicely browned.

In a separate bowl, combine the courgette ribbons with the chopped tomatoes, parsley and mint and mix together. Place on a serving platter, pile the cooked meatballs on top and drizzle over the dressing.

Seared Steaks with Roasted Pepper and Almond Sauce

Serves 4
Contains nuts
—

4 rump or sirloin steaks,
   each 3–4cm/
   1¼–1½in thick
1 tbsp olive oil

For the sauce
½ tbsp olive oil
4 red peppers
25g/1oz flaked almonds
1 large tomato
Sea salt and freshly
   ground black pepper

This combination of peppers, almonds and beef is divine, although the better the quality of beef you use, the more fabulous it will taste. I always buy organic beef as the flavour is far superior; I would rather eat less meat and make sure it is organic. Try to use a griddle pan to cook the steak (a barbeque would be even better) and then serve cut into slices with a bowl of the dip and perhaps my Potatoes with Parsley, Capers and Lemon (see page 104) to accompany it. I like steak served rare, so I have included the appropriate cooking times. If you prefer your steak medium, then sear for 3–4 minutes each side before leaving to rest.

Preheat the oven to 220°C/425°F/gas mark 7.

Begin by making the sauce. Rub the olive oil over the peppers, then place on a baking tray and roast in the oven for 35 minutes or until softened and slightly charred. Remove from the oven and place in a plastic freezer or storage bag. Seal and leave for approximately 30 minutes, then take out of the bag and carefully peel off the skins, cut out the stalks and remove the seeds.

Meanwhile, scatter the flaked almonds on a baking tray and toast in the oven, turning them from time to time to make sure they don't burn, for 5–6 minutes or until golden. Remove and set aside to cool.

Roughly chop the tomato and add to a food processor or blender with the roasted peppers and flaked almonds. Season well with salt and pepper and blitz until completely smooth, then transfer to bowl and chill in the fridge for 30 minutes before serving.

Remove the steaks from the fridge 20 minutes or so before cooking them, to bring them up to room temperature, and rub them with the olive oil. Heat a griddle pan or heavy-based frying pan over a high heat for 5–10 minutes (you want the pan to be searing hot) and then add the steaks. Sear for 2½ minutes on one side without touching it, then turn over and sear for another 2–3 minutes. Remove from the heat and leave to rest for 10 minutes.

When ready to serve, slice widthways into strips approximately 2.5cm/1in thick. Serve with individual bowls of the pepper and almond sauce on the side.

Penne with Fennel and Salami

Serves 4
Contains nuts
—

25g/1oz pine nuts
2 large fennel bulbs
200g/7oz piece of salami
2 cloves of garlic
1kg/2lb 3oz ripe plum
   tomatoes
2 tbsp olive oil
1 tsp chilli flakes
400g/14oz gluten-free
   penne
A bunch of flat-leaf
   parsley
Sea salt and freshly
   ground black pepper

I have to admit to having a real passion for fennel. Here its pungent aniseed flavour really counterbalances the robust taste of the salami, making for a wonderfully rich pasta dish. You will need a block or 'round' of salami for this recipe – fairly easy to find in good delis or, indeed, the deli counter in big supermarkets. Do be aware, though, that a number of salamis contain lactose or wheat in some form, so check the ingredients first to be sure. There are many different types of salami so just choose your favourite kind, although I do favour the slightly denser German variety.

In a heavy-based frying pan, dry-fry the pine nuts over a medium–high heat for 3–4 minutes or until golden, shaking the pan regularly to ensure that they don't burn. Remove from the heat and allow to cool.

Trim the fennel bulbs, remove the outer leaves, cut in half lengthways and finely slice. Cut the salami into thin strips approximately 6cm/2½in long and 5mm/¼in wide and finely slice the garlic into rounds.

Next skin the tomatoes. Place in a large bowl, cover with boiling water and leave for 1 minute. Drain the tomatoes and carefully peel away the skins (they should slide off with ease), then slice in half and scoop out the seeds. Roughly chop the flesh and set aside.

Add the olive oil to a heavy-based saucepan on a low heat, tip in the salami and the sliced garlic and gently fry for 1 minute – the salami should release some of its oil and start to become deeper in colour. Add the sliced fennel to the pan, turn the heat up a little, cover with a lid and cook for a further 5 minutes, stirring once or twice to make sure the fennel and garlic don't catch on the base of the pan.

Add the chopped tomatoes and the chilli flakes and season well with salt and pepper. Bring the sauce to a gentle simmer, then cover with a lid and cook for 20 minutes or until the sauce has thickened and the fennel is cooked through.

Meanwhile, bring a large saucepan of salted water to the boil, add the penne and cook until al dente following the instructions on the packet – usually 10–12 minutes, depending on the brand of pasta. Once cooked, drain and return to the empty pan. Pour over the fennel and salami sauce and stir into the penne. Spoon into bowls, then finely chop the parsley and scatter both this and the toasted pine nuts over the pasta to serve.

Summer Tomato and Pesto Tart

Serves 8
Contains nuts
—

2 red onions
5 large vine-ripened
   tomatoes
4 tbsp olive oil
1 tsp soft light brown
   sugar
1 quantity of Shortcrust
   Pastry (see page 223)
Sea salt and freshly
   ground black pepper

For the pesto
50g/1¾oz pine nuts
Leaves from a bunch
   of basil
1½ tbsp extra-virgin
   olive oil
Sea salt and freshly
   ground black pepper

You will need a 23cm/9in diameter tart tin with a removable base for this recipe

This is a wonderful savoury tart to serve, hot or cold, for a summer lunch or picnic. The shortcrust pastry provides a buttery base for the sweet and juicy tomatoes, while the pesto adds warmth and fragrance.

Preheat the oven to 190°C/375°C/gas mark 5.

First make the pesto. Scatter the pine nuts on a baking tray and toast in the oven, turning occasionally to make sure they don't burn, for 5–6 minutes or until golden brown, then remove and set aside to cool.

Finely chop the basil and mix with the toasted pine nuts and olive oil, then, using a pestle and mortar, pound them together until smooth. Season with salt and pepper to taste and add a little more olive oil if you think it's necessary. Alternatively, add the toasted pine nuts to a food processor and blitz to a fine-breadcrumb consistency. Add the basil and seasoning and pour over the olive oil, then blitz until you have a smooth paste.

Next, halve the onions and slice into thin half-moons. Trim the ends from each tomato and slice into rounds approximately 5mm/¼in thick. Heat 3 tablespoons of the olive oil in a non-stick frying pan and add the onions. Sauté over a low heat for about 20 minutes or until completely softened but not browned, adding the sugar and seasoning with salt and pepper halfway through cooking.

Meanwhile, roll out the pastry and fill the tart tin following the instructions given in the Shortcrust Pastry recipe on page 223.

Spread the caramelised onions over the base of the tart and then add small dollops of the pesto, spaced evenly apart, on top of the onions. Layer the tomatoes into the tart in a circular pattern, allowing them to overlap slightly. Drizzle with the remaining oil, season well with salt and pepper and bake in the oven for 35–40 minutes. Remove from the oven and allow to cool for around 5 minutes before carefully removing the tart from its tin and cutting into slices.

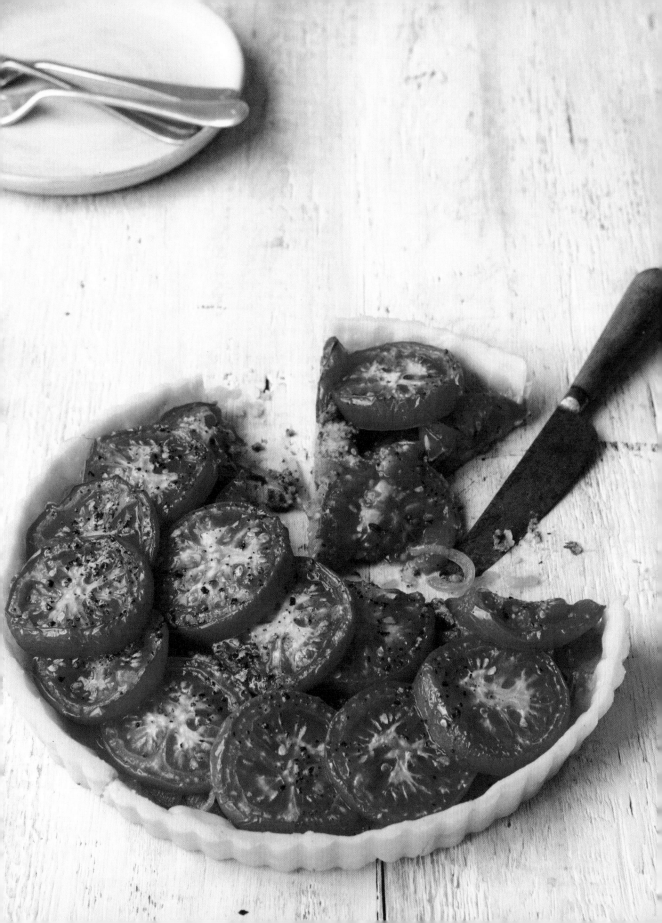

Roasted Tomatoes, Butterbeans and Sweet Peppers with Thyme

Serves 4

—

250g/9oz butterbeans
6 plum tomatoes
2 red peppers
1 orange pepper
4 tbsp olive oil
2 tsp soft light brown
    sugar
6 sprigs of thyme
Sea salt and freshly
    ground black pepper

This ultra-simple dish is nonetheless packed full of flavour and perfect for a relaxed lunch or supper. The sweetness of the tomatoes and peppers is offset by the beans, which develop a golden crust on top while remaining soft and creamy in the middle. I like to serve this with a little cooked quinoa with handfuls of fresh, mixed herbs chopped up and folded in. I recommend cooking the butterbeans yourself as this really adds to the texture and flavour of the dish; but feel free to use a good-quality tinned variety if you don't have the time.

Prepare the beans by placing them in a large saucepan, covering with plenty of water (don't add salt at this point as it can make the skins of the beans tough). Bring to the boil and then remove from the heat and leave to soak for 1½ hours. Drain the beans and rinse under cold water before setting aside.

Preheat the oven to 200°C/400°F/gas mark 6.

Next, halve the tomatoes and prepare the peppers by slicing them in half lengthways and removing the stalks and seeds before cutting into lengths approximately 2cm/¾in thick.

Spread the peppers and tomatoes out in a large roasting tin and scatter the cooked butterbeans among them. Drizzle with the olive oil, sprinkle over the sugar and add the sprigs of thyme. Bake in the oven for 50–55 minutes, giving the pan a shake occasionally, then remove from the oven, discarding the thyme, and season well with salt and pepper before serving.

Ratatouille

Serves 4

—

1 yellow pepper
1 red pepper
1 aubergine
1 red onion
2 cloves of garlic
2 courgettes
2 tbsp olive oil
A large bunch of basil
A small bunch of oregano
500ml/18fl oz passata
200g/7oz sun-blushed
   tomatoes
1 tsp soft light brown
   sugar
2 tsp lemon juice
Sea salt and freshly
   ground black pepper

So simple and a joy to make, this is the perfect all-round vegetarian dish. Delicious and highly versatile, it can be served hot or cold, either on its own with rice or used for stuffing peppers, filling a baked potato or as a base for lasagne or other pasta dishes. It is also particularly handy for using up gluts of vegetables, so feel free to vary the ingredients depending on what you may have in your fridge or garden – I often add fennel, sweet potatoes or green beans to the mix.

Preheat the oven to 200°C/400°F/gas mark 6.

Deseed the peppers and cut these and the aubergine and onion into 2cm/¾in cubes. Crush the garlic, then halve the courgettes lengthways and cut into half-moons about 1cm/½in thick.

Combine all the vegetables in a large roasting tin, pour over the olive oil and mix well, then roast in the oven for around 40 minutes or until all the vegetables are tender and just starting to caramelise at the edges.

Finely chop the basil and oregano and add to a large saucepan with the passata, sun-blushed tomatoes, sugar and lemon juice, before stirring in the roasted vegetables and seasoning with salt and pepper. Bring to a simmer, then cover and cook very gently for 15 minutes before serving.

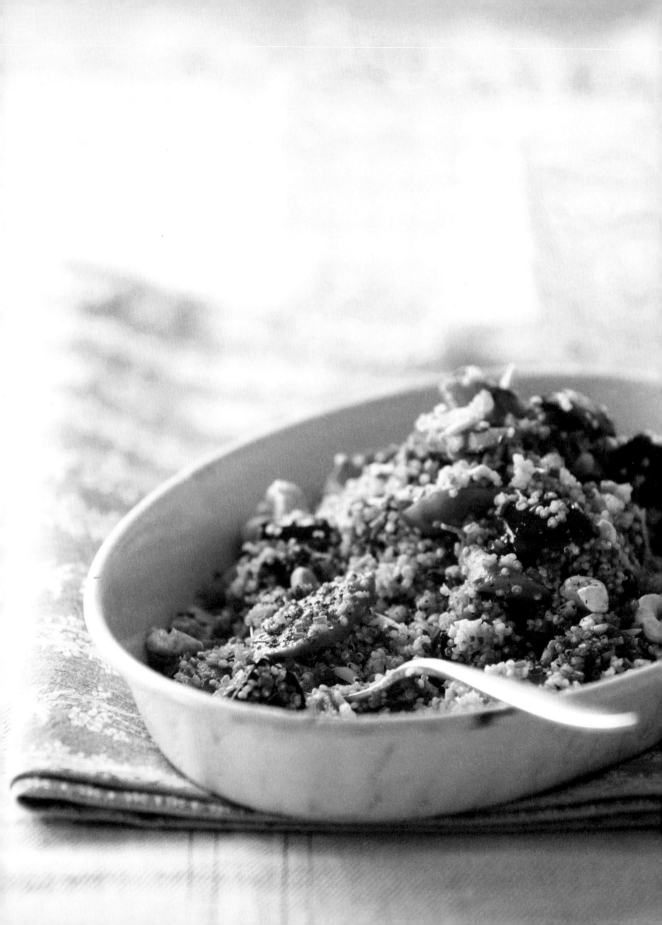

Roasted Aubergine and Quinoa Salad

Serves 4
Contains nuts
—
175g/6oz quinoa
500ml/18fl oz vegetable
   stock
3 large carrots
1 aubergine
½ tsp cumin seeds
¼ tsp coriander seeds
½ tsp ground cinnamon
1 tbsp runny honey
3 tbsp olive oil
30g/1¼oz unsalted
   cashew nuts
A bunch of chives
Grated zest and juice
   of 1 lemon
Sea salt and freshly
   ground black pepper

Ancient in origin, quinoa is not only a superfood, packed with nutrients, but utterly delicious. My favourite use for the grain is as part of a fragrant, colourful salad; its ability to absorb and boost flavours makes it the ideal base. Here, the nutty quinoa mingles with sweet, roasted carrot, mellow, smoky aubergine and a delicate blend of spices, while the toasted cashews and fresh chives add bite and a lively contrast.

Place the quinoa in a large saucepan and pour over the stock, then cover with a lid and bring to the boil. Once boiling, reduce the heat to low and simmer gently for about 15 minutes or until the quinoa has absorbed all of the stock. Fluff the cooked quinoa with a fork and then set aside while you prepare the vegetables.

Preheat the oven to 220°C/425°F/gas mark 7.

Cut the carrots into 5mm/½in rounds and the aubergine into 1.5cm/⅝in cubes. Using a pestle and mortar, grind the cumin and coriander seeds into a fine powder or place in a plastic bag and crush with a rolling pin.

Place the carrots and aubergine in a large roasting tin and combine with the freshly ground spices, cinnamon, honey and olive oil. Season well with salt and pepper and cover the tin tightly with foil before roasting in the oven for 15 minutes. Remove the foil and continue to roast for a further 5 minutes.

Meanwhile, scatter the cashew nuts on a baking tray and toast in the oven, turning them occasionally to make sure they don't burn, for 5–6 minutes or until golden brown, then remove and allow to cool. Finally chop the chives and set aside.

Combine the quinoa with the roasted vegetables, lemon zest and toasted cashews. Then fold in the lemon juice and chopped chives, season with salt and pepper to taste and serve while the vegetables are still warm.

Warm Lentil Salad with Roasted Fennel and Sun-blushed Tomatoes

Serves 4
Contains nuts

—

50g/1¾oz shelled
    hazelnuts
2 cloves of garlic
2 fennel bulbs
250g/9oz Puy lentils
1 tbsp olive oil
A small bunch of
    curly-leaf parsley
150g/5oz sun-blushed
    tomatoes
Sea salt and freshly
    ground black pepper

For the dressing
2 tbsp extra-virgin
    olive oil
1 tbsp lemon juice
2 tsp agave syrup
Sea salt and freshly
    ground black pepper

This salad is a wonderful medley of taste and colour, the aniseed flavour of the roasted fennel combining with the sweet intensity of the sun-blushed tomatoes, while the toasted hazelnuts add a buttery bite. Be sure to use a really good-quality olive oil for the dressing; it makes all the difference to the flavour and adds a glorious sheen to the cooked lentils. I like to serve this warm – or, at a push, at room temperature – with a leafy green salad or a handful of baby-leaf spinach on the side.

Preheat the oven to 200°C/400°F/gas mark 6.

Scatter the hazelnuts on a baking tray and toast in the oven, turning them occasionally to make sure they don't burn, for 5–6 minutes or until golden brown, then remove and set aside to cool.

Meanwhile, crush the garlic and then trim the fennel bulbs and cut into quarters, slicing each quarter into 1.5cm/⅝in chunks.

Place the lentils in a large saucepan and pour over enough water to cover them to a depth of at least 8cm/3in. Bring to the boil, then reduce the heat to low and simmer for 20–25 minutes or until the lentils are just tender, adding more water during cooking if necessary.

Meanwhile, place the fennel in a roasting tin and combine with the garlic and olive oil. Season well with salt and pepper and roast in the oven for 20 minutes or until the fennel is tender and golden at the edges. Once cooked, remove from the oven and set aside.

In a small bowl, mix together all the ingredients for the dressing, seasoning well with salt and pepper and whisking with a fork to amalgamate the flavours.

Once the lentils are cooked, drain in a colander and tip into a serving bowl. Pour over the dressing, then stir well, seasoning to taste and adding more olive oil if you think it needs it. Finely chop the parsley and add to the lentils with the roasted fennel, sun-blushed tomatoes and toasted hazelnuts, mix together and serve while warm.

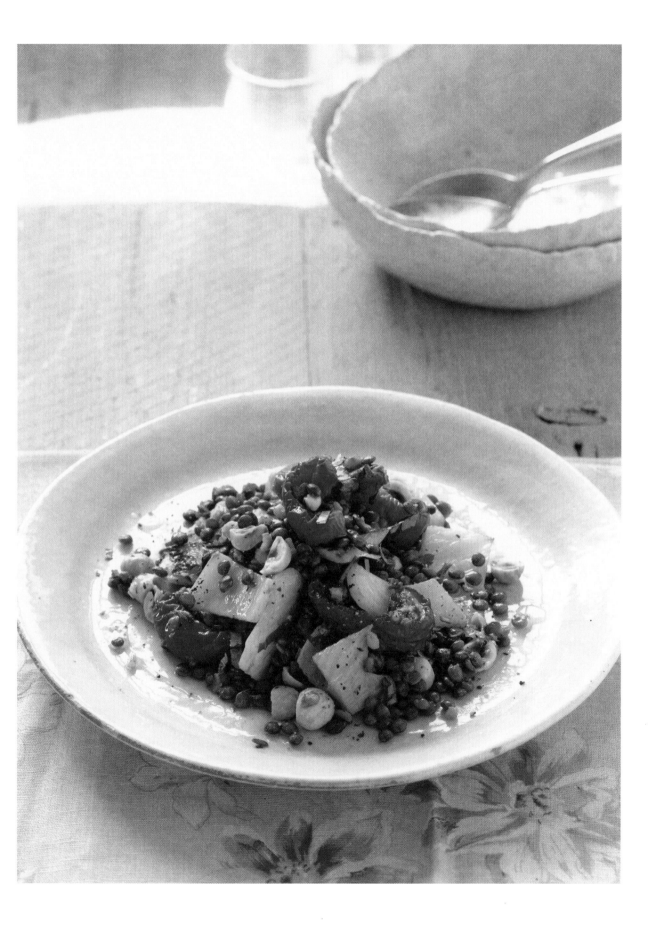

Potatoes with Parsley, Capers and Lemon

Serves 4

—

1kg/2lb 3oz floury potatoes
  (ideally Maris Piper
  or Lady Balfour)
4 tbsp olive oil
A bunch of flat-leaf parsley
2 tbsp capers, drained
  and rinsed
Grated zest and juice
  of 1 lemon
Sea salt and freshly
  ground black pepper

Crisp and packed full of flavour, these potatoes make a glorious accompaniment to roasted meats or to serve alongside grilled prawns, seared salmon, roasted peppers or even a slow-cooked stew. I recommend using Maris Piper or Lady Balfour potatoes as they crunch up particularly well.

Preheat the oven to 200°C/400°F/gas mark 6.

Peel the potatoes and cut into 2cm/¾in cubes. Place in a large, non-stick roasting tin, then add half the olive oil, season well with salt and pepper and mix together, ensuring that the potatoes are spread evenly in the tin and not piled on top of each other.

Place in the oven and roast for 35–45 minutes, turning them halfway through cooking, until crisp and golden brown. Remove from the oven and, while hot, transfer to a serving dish. Roughly chop the parsley and add to the roasted potatoes with the remaining olive oil, capers and lemon zest and juice. Season again with salt and pepper and mix together thoroughly. Serve immediately.

Tomato, Basil and Pine Nut Quinoa

Serves 4
Contains nuts

—

25g/1oz pine nuts
175g/6oz quinoa
500ml/18fl oz vegetable
  stock
½ quantity of Slow-
  roasted Tomatoes
  (see page 172)
A small bunch of basil

This is a versatile dish that can be served as a salad, either warm or cold, or used for stuffing peppers and courgettes. Or just serve on its own with a large dollop of houmous. If you don't have the time or the inclination to make the slow-roasted tomatoes, then sun-blushed tomatoes will do just as well.

In a heavy-based frying pan, dry-fry the pine nuts over a medium–high heat for 3–4 minutes or until golden, shaking the pan regularly to ensure that they don't burn. Remove from the heat and set aside to cool.

Place the quinoa in a large saucepan and pour over the stock, then cover with a lid and bring to the boil. Once boiling, reduce the heat to low and simmer gently for about 15 minutes or until the quinoa has absorbed all of the stock. Remove from the heat and fluff up the cooked grains with a fork.

Finely slice the slow-roasted tomatoes and the basil and stir into the quinoa before scattering over the toasted pine nuts to serve.

Pesto New Potato Salad

Serves 4
Contains nuts

—

100g/3½oz pine nuts
Leaves from a large
   bunch of basil
3 tbsp extra-virgin olive oil
450g/1lb new potatoes
   (unpeeled)
Sea salt and freshly
   ground black pepper

This salad sounds incredibly simple and indeed it is, but no less appetising for it. In fact, its simplicity is its secret weapon. With so few ingredients, the flavours stand proud and demand to be noticed, and when you are using fresh, high-quality produce, it makes sense to keep the fuss to a minimum and let the food do the talking. I love this pesto; by toasting the pine nuts first, they take on a little of the nutty intensity of Parmesan cheese, lending the pesto a moreish flavour that makes you want to serve it with everything. The options are endless, but this salad is one of my favourite ways of using the pesto, which is absorbed by the steaming hot potatoes, their tender, creamy flesh yielding a layer of nutty, salty pesto when you bite into them. Sheer bliss!

In a heavy-based frying pan, dry-fry the pine nuts over a medium–high heat for 3–4 minutes or until golden, shaking the pan regularly to ensure that they don't burn. Remove from the heat and allow to cool.

Finely chop the basil and mix with the toasted pine nuts and olive oil, then, using a pestle and mortar, pound them together until smooth. Season with salt and pepper to taste and add a little more olive oil if you think it's necessary. Alternatively, add the toasted pine nuts to a food processor and blitz until a fine-breadcrumb consistency. Add the basil and seasoning and pour over the olive oil, then blitz until you have a smooth paste.

Bring a large pan of salted water to the boil and add the new potatoes. (A tip worth knowing is to always add new potatoes to boiling water, whereas old potatoes should be placed in the water when cold and then brought to the boil.) Cook for 15–20 minutes or until completely tender when tested with the point of a knife. Drain in a colander and, while hot, fold in the fresh pesto to serve.

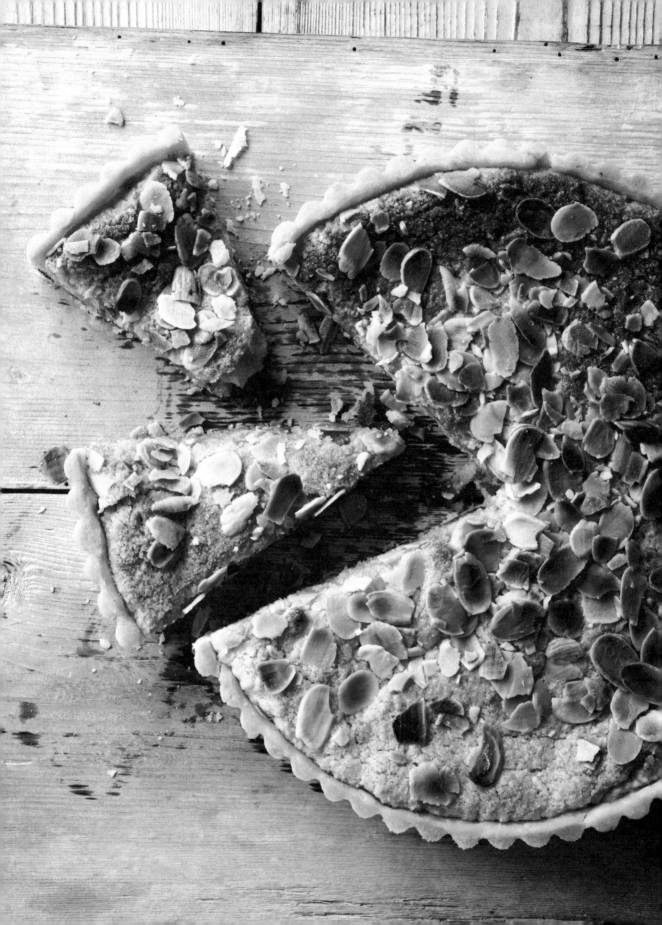

Bakewell Tart

Serves 8
Contains nuts

—

1 quantity of sweet
  Shortcrust Pastry
  (see page 223)

For the jam filling
150g/5oz fresh raspberries
1½ tbsp golden caster
  sugar

For the almond filling
150g/5oz Pure
  Sunflower Spread
  (dairy-free margarine)
150g/5oz golden caster
  sugar
2 heaped tsp egg replacer
  (ideally Orgran) whisked
  with 4 tbsp water
100g/3½oz ground rice
200g/7oz ground almonds
¼ tsp almond extract
A large handful of flaked
  almonds

*You will need a 23cm/9in
diameter tart tin with
a removable base for
this recipe*

Bakewell tart has always held a special place in my heart. I love the glorious combination of buttery almond filling, shortcrust pastry and sharply sweet raspberry jam. When I first discovered that I could no longer eat wheat, dairy produce and eggs, I was certain that I would have to say goodbye to the crumbly deliciousness that is Bakewell tart. Not so: in fact, this recipe is so close to the real deal that it may even outdo it! Serve it to your friends and family and, most importantly, tuck into a slice yourself – you'll be over the moon, I guarantee it.

First make the jam filling. Place the raspberries and caster sugar in a small saucepan over a low heat. Heat gently for about 10 minutes, allowing the berries to slowly break down and reduce to a jammy consistency, then set aside to cool.

Next make the almond filling. Cream the margarine and sugar together gently with a wooden spoon until pale and fluffy. Add the egg replacer mixture, bit by bit and stirring as you go until fully combined, then stir in the ground rice, ground almonds and almond extract.

Preheat the oven to 190°C/375°F/gas mark 5.

Roll out the pastry and fill the tart tin following the instructions given in the Shortcrust Pastry recipe on page 223.

Spread the base of the tart with the raspberry jam and then carefully spoon over the almond filling, smoothing the top into one even layer using the back of a spoon. Scatter over the flaked almonds and bake in the oven for 35–40 minutes or until golden on top. Serve on its own, cooled down, or still warm with a scoop of Vanilla Ice Cream (see page 66) on the side.

Strawberry and Lime Sorbet

Serves 6

—

225g/8oz golden caster
    sugar
2 tbsp agave syrup
1kg/2lb 3oz ripe
    strawberries
4 tbsp lime juice

*You will need an ice-cream
maker (minimum capacity
of 1 litre/1¾ pints) for this
recipe if not making the
sorbet by hand*

This sorbet is everything you could ask for: sweet and sharp, crisp and creamy, cool and comforting. Whether you have an ice-cream maker or not, you really must try this – it is summertime in a bowl.

Place the sugar in a saucepan and pour over 225ml/8fl oz of water, then set over a low heat and stir to dissolve the sugar. Bring to the boil and as soon as the mixture starts to boil, remove from the heat and set aside to cool. (You could prepare this syrup up to a week in advance, storing it in a jar in your fridge ready to use on the day.)

Place the sugar syrup and agave syrup in a saucepan and boil for 5 minutes, then remove from the heat and allow it to cool. Meanwhile, hull the strawberries and purée with the lime juice in a food processor or blender. Pass the strawberry purée through a sieve, discarding the pips. Once the syrup is cool, mix it into the strawberry purée and immediately transfer to an ice-cream maker to churn for 20–30 minutes.

Alternatively, you can make the sorbet by hand. Pour the mixture into a freezer-proof container or plastic tub and freeze for 1 hour or until solid, remove from the freezer, cut into rough chunks and, using a hand-held blender or a food processor, blitz until smooth.

Once the sorbet is made (whether in the ice-cream maker or by hand), pour into a freezer-proof container, cover with cling film and freeze for at least 3 hours before serving.

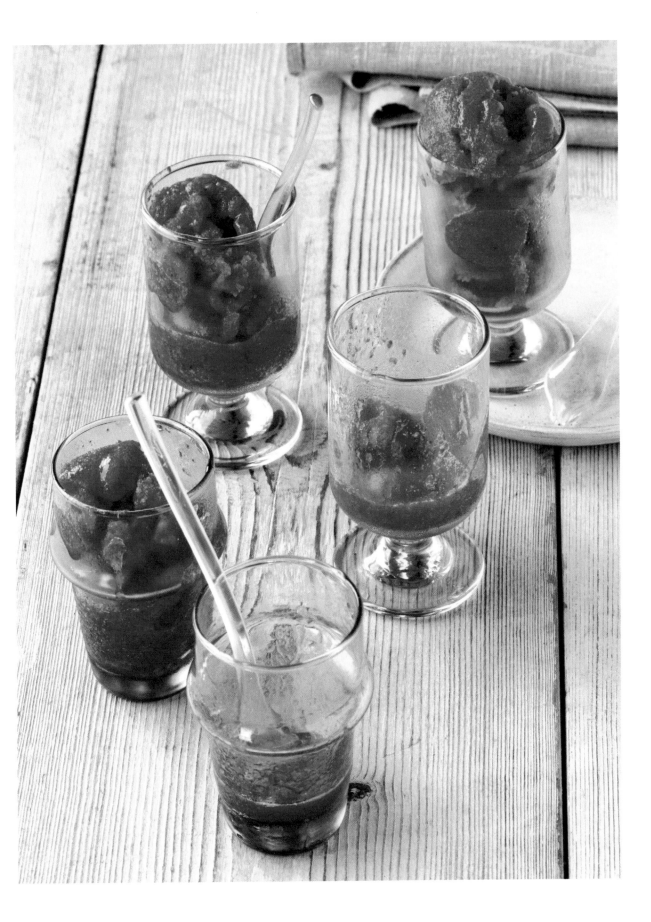

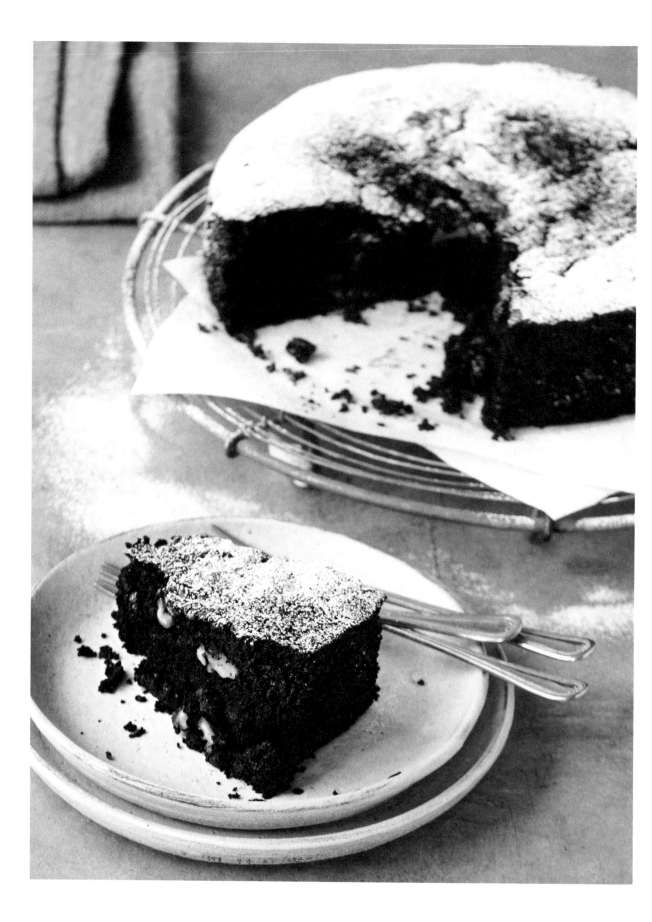

Mocha Fudge Cake

Serves 8
Contains nuts

—

100g/3½fl oz rapeseed
  oil, plus extra for
  greasing
50g/1¾oz shelled
  walnuts
200g/7oz gluten-free
  plain flour (ideally
  Doves Farm)
50g/1¾oz cocoa powder
1 tsp baking powder
1½ tsp bicarbonate
  of soda
A pinch of sea salt
300ml/10½fl oz maple
  syrup
110ml/4fl oz rice milk
100ml/3½fl oz freshly
  made coffee
Icing sugar, for dusting

You will need a 20cm/
8in diameter cake tin
with a removable base
for this recipe

Here, the rich taste of chocolate melds with the bitter bite of coffee to create
a divine treat for serving with an afternoon cup of tea or as an indulgent
dessert. Don't be put off by how liquid the batter appears initially – it is this
that gives the cake such a wonderful, gooey texture. As to the type of coffee:
you can use fully caffeinated or decaf, depending on your whim.

Preheat the oven to 170°C/325°F/gas mark 3, then lightly grease
the cake tin and line the base with baking parchment.

Scatter the walnuts on a baking tray and toast in the oven, turning
occasionally to make sure they don't burn, for 5–8 minutes or until
lightly browned, then remove and allow to cool before chopping into
small pieces.

Next, sift the flour into a large bowl with the cocoa powder, baking
powder, bicarbonate of soda and salt. In a separate bowl, whisk together
the maple syrup, rice milk, coffee and rapeseed oil until combined. Pour
the liquid ingredients into the flour mixture and beat together until
smooth, then stir in the chopped walnuts.

Pour the batter into the prepared tin and bake in the oven for
40–45 minutes or until risen and springy to a light touch. If in doubt,
insert a skewer or cocktail stick into the centre of the cake – if it comes
out clean, then it is cooked. Remove from the oven and transfer the tin
to a wire rack, allowing the cake to cool completely before dusting with
icing sugar and cutting into slices to serve.

Carrot Cake with Lemon Fudge Icing

Serves 8–10
Contains nuts
—

150g/5oz Pure Sunflower Spread (dairy-free margarine), plus extra for greasing
150g/5oz soft dark brown sugar
2 heaped tsp egg replacer (ideally Orgran) whisked with 4 tbsp water
150g/5oz trimmed, peeled and grated carrots
150g/5oz gluten-free self-raising flour (ideally Doves Farm)
1 tsp mixed spice
60g/2oz ground almonds

For the lemon icing
60g/2oz Pure Sunflower Spread (dairy-free margarine)
Grated zest of 1 lemon and 2 tbsp lemon juice
225g/8oz icing sugar, sifted

You will need two 20cm/ 8in diameter sandwich tins for this recipe

A delicious combination of sweetly moist carrots, mellow mixed spice and fluffy ground almonds with the bright citrus tang of the lemon butter cream icing, this cake is perfect for afternoon tea. It's best to grate the carrots by hand rather than using a food processor as this produces a lot of excess water, making your cake soggy. You could also bake it into a Carrot Traybake: tip the batter into a lined 18 x 28cm/7 x 11in tin and bake for 35–40 minutes before smothering with the lemon icing and cutting into slices. If you store it in the fridge, covered in cling film, the cake will keep for up to four days.

Preheat the oven to 190°C/375°F/gas mark 5, then lightly grease the sandwich tins and line the bases with baking parchment.

In a large bowl, cream together the sugar and margarine gently with a wooden spoon until thick and fluffy, then stir in the egg replacer mixture, bit by bit and beating as you go. Stir in the grated carrots, then sift in the flour and mixed spice, folding it in with the ground almonds until all the ingredients are combined.

Spoon the cake mixture into the prepared tins, spreading it out to the edges and levelling the top with the back of a spoon, then bake in the oven for 17–20 minutes or until golden and slightly springy to a light touch. Remove from the oven and leave in the tins for a few minutes before turning out onto a wire rack and leaving to cool completely.

Meanwhile, make the icing. Melt the margarine with the lemon juice and zest in a small saucepan over a low heat, then remove from the heat and vigorously stir in the icing sugar until the mixture is smooth, glossy and thick. Once the cake has cooled completely, spread three-quarters of the icing over one of the cakes and then gently rest the remaining cake on top. Spread the rest of the icing over the top. Cut into slices to serve.

Chocolate Ice Cream

Serves 4

—

350ml/12fl oz almond
   or oat milk
250ml/9fl oz oat cream
50g/1¾oz golden
   caster sugar
2½ tbsp cocoa powder

*You will need an ice-cream
maker (minimum capacity
of 1 litre/1¾ pints) for
this recipe if not making
the ice cream by hand*

*Nothing says summertime more than a bowl of creamy, sweet ice cream.
Although it may not be the first thing that springs to mind when you think
of allergy-friendly cooking, I promise you that once you have made this, you
will never look back. I find the best way to prepare ice cream is to use an
ice-cream maker as this always produces the perfect consistency, but you
can of course make it by hand if you prefer.*

Place the almond or oat milk in a large saucepan with the oat cream
and sugar and set over a medium heat, whisking constantly, until the
sugar has completely dissolved.

Place the cocoa powder in a bowl and pour over a little bit of the
hot milk. Mix into a smooth paste before slowly pouring into the hot
milk in the pan, then whisk until smooth.

Set the mixture aside to cool down. Once cool, refrigerate for
10 minutes before pouring into the ice-cream maker and churning for
20–30 minutes. (Keep an eye on the ice cream while it is churning to
catch it when it has become creamy and smooth in consistency, just
past being 'soft set'.)

To make the ice cream by hand, pour the cooled mixture into a
freezer-proof container or plastic tub and freeze for 1 hour or until
solid. Remove from the freezer, cut into rough chunks and, using a
hand-held blender or a food processor, blitz until smooth. Place the ice
cream in the fridge and leave for a further hour before blitzing again.

Once the ice cream is made (whether in the ice-cream maker or
by hand), it can be served immediately for soft-set ice cream or,
alternatively, poured into a freezer-proof container, covered with
cling film and frozen for at least 3 hours before serving.

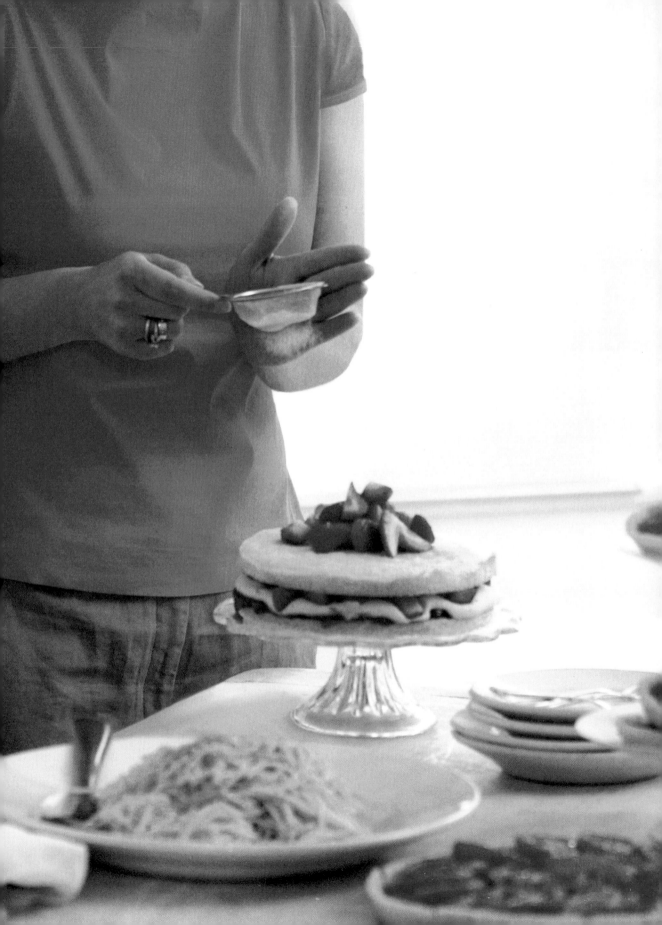

Victoria Sponge with Strawberries and Vanilla Cream

Serves 8
Contains nuts
—

175g/6oz Pure
   Sunflower Spread
   (dairy-free margarine),
   plus extra for greasing
175g/6oz golden caster
   sugar
A few drops of vanilla
   extract
2 heaped tsp egg replacer
   (ideally Orgran) whisked
   with 4 tbsp water
175g/6oz gluten-free plain
   flour (ideally Doves Farm)
1 tsp baking powder
¼ tsp xanthan gum
1½ tbsp rice milk
Icing sugar, for dusting

For the filling
100g/3½oz fresh
   strawberries
2 tbsp strawberry jam

For the vanilla cream
200g/7oz unsalted
   cashew nuts
150ml/5fl oz almond milk
1 tsp agave syrup
¼ tsp vanilla extract
Seeds from 1 vanilla pod

You will need two 20cm/8in
diameter sandwich tins for
this recipe

This cake is a true British classic – rich with jam, cream and fresh, sweet fruit – but with an ingenious vegan twist. Instead of conventional dairy-based cream I've used a combination of raw cashew nuts and almond milk to make a luxuriant and smooth vanilla cream with a light vanilla flavour. It pays to make the vanilla cream in advance as it needs to be chilled in the fridge in order to thicken up and hold its shape. Once made, it will keep, covered, in the fridge for up to a week and can be used to serve with all sorts of puddings, from simple strawberries and cream to Bakewell Tart or Chocolate Nut Brownies (see pages 107 and 63).

Begin by making the vanilla cream. Place the cashew nuts in a blender or food processor with the almond milk, agave syrup and vanilla extract, and pulse until smooth, thick and creamy – if you feel like the mixture is too grainy, just continue to blitz until smooth, adding a little extra almond milk as you go. Stir in the seeds from the vanilla pod, then transfer to a bowl, cover and chill in the fridge for 1–2 hours.

Preheat the oven to 190°C/375°F/gas mark 5, then grease the sandwich tins and line the bases with baking parchment.

Lightly cream together the margarine, caster sugar and vanilla extract with a wooden spoon until incorporated. Stir in the egg replacer mixture, bit by bit, until fully combined (don't worry if the batter looks a little curdled at this point – the flour will pull it back together). Sift in the flour, baking powder and xanthan gum, add the rice milk and stir until you have a smooth batter.

Divide the mixture between the prepared tins and bake in the oven, on the middle shelf, for 15–20 minutes or until the cake is springy to a light touch. Remove from the oven and carefully turn out onto a wire rack to cool completely.

While the cakes are cooling, hull the strawberries and cut into quarters. Spread the strawberry jam over the top of one of the cooled cakes and then carefully spoon over the vanilla cream. Scatter over the strawberries and top with the second cake. Sift over a little icing sugar and cut into slices to serve.

Blueberry Shortcake Biscuits

Makes about 12 biscuits

—

110g/4oz gluten-free plain flour (ideally Doves Farm)

1 tsp baking powder

A small pinch of sea salt

30g/1¼oz golden caster sugar

75g/3oz Pure Sunflower Spread (dairy-free margarine)

125ml/4½fl oz oat cream

½ tsp lemon juice

170g/6oz fresh blueberries

Calling these 'biscuits' is perhaps a bit misleading – in density and texture, they are more like scones, enlivened by the fresh burst of blueberry as you bite into them. Crying out to be served with a cup of tea in the afternoon, they will feel like a real treat whatever the occasion. I would recommend that you eat them on the day of making as the oat cream in the mixture causes them to go soft very quickly. All the more reason to help yourself to another one!

Preheat the oven to 190°C/375°F/gas mark 5 and line a large baking sheet with baking parchment.

Sift the flour into a large bowl with the baking powder and salt and stir in the sugar. Cut the margarine into small pieces and rub into the flour until the mixture resembles coarse breadcrumbs. Stir in the oat cream and lemon juice until the mixture starts to come together, then add the blueberries and stir gently until combined.

Using a tablespoon, drop spoonfuls of the shortbread mixture onto the baking sheet, then use the back of the spoon to shape each biscuit into a circle approximately 5cm/2in in diameter, spacing them evenly apart.

Bake for 35–40 minutes or until golden brown, then remove and allow to cool for 5 minutes before carefully lifting from the baking parchment and transferring to a wire rack to cool completely.

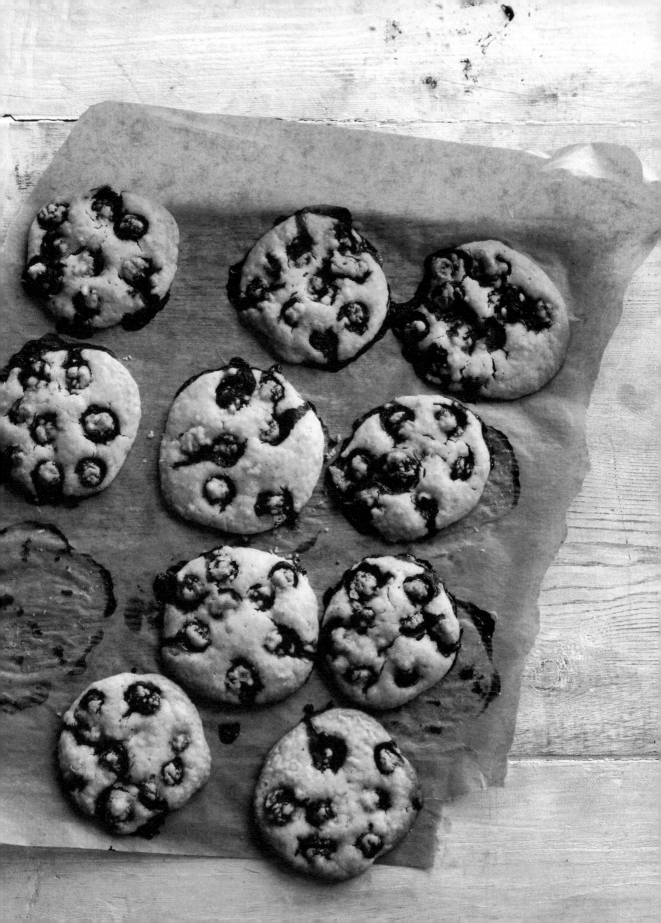

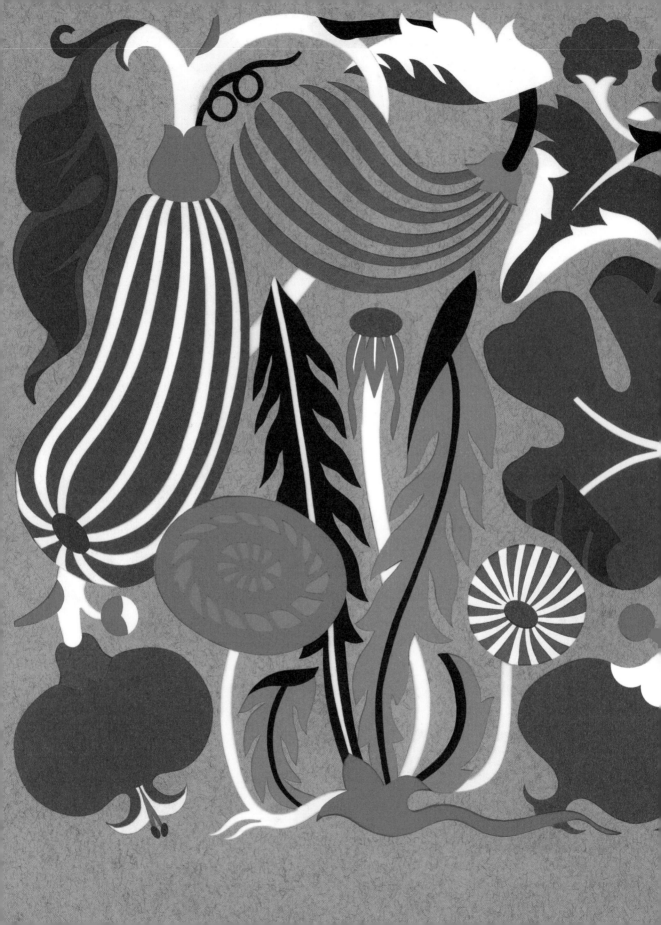

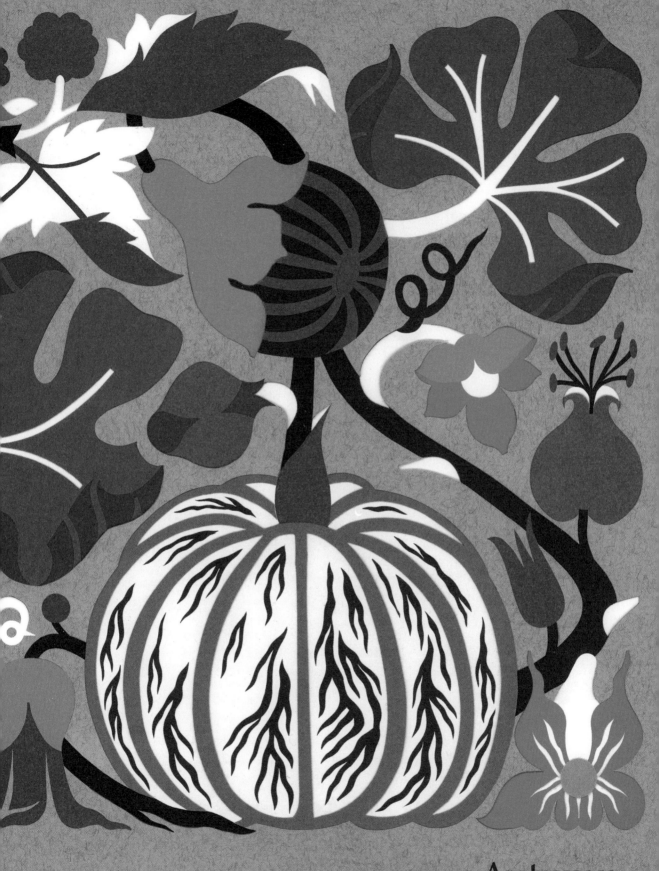

Autumn

Autumnal food should be rich and ample, spiked with woody herbs and warming spices. Butternut squash, mushrooms, apples and plums all come into their own, adding mellow flavour and satisfying texture, while slow-baked dishes and savoury roasts are the order of the day. Recipes such as the Sweet Potato, Thyme and Bacon Tartlets (see page 125) offer a light meal on just the right side of simple and packed full of smoky and aromatic flavour. Spaghetti Carbonara (see page 142) will wrap you in creamy comfort with a delicately nutty edge – perfect for sharing with friends and family on a chilly evening, while Sticky Date Squares (see page 163) provide the sweetest of treats, merging crumbly, buttery oats with a glorious layer of melted, sugary dates, guaranteed to warm the soul.

Cream of Chicken and Mushroom Soup

Serves 4

—

2 tbsp olive oil

1 large white onion

500g/1lb 2oz chestnut mushrooms

1.2 litres/2 pints chicken stock

A small bunch of marjoram

Leaves from 4 sprigs of thyme

400g/14oz cooked chicken

110ml/4fl oz oat cream

A small bunch of curly-leaf parsley

Sea salt and freshly ground black pepper

A hearty, warming bowlful – perfect for those autumnal days when you need both comfort and sustenance. I think of this as a meal in itself and needs little accompaniment other than perhaps an extra sprinkling of chopped parsley and a slice of Rye Soda Bread (see page 214). Saying that, for an instant supper, I have on occasion poured a ladleful of this soup over a bowl of pasta, with lovely results. This is a great soup to make when using up leftover roast chicken – finely dice the remaining meat and make the chicken stock from the leftover carcass.

Pour the olive oil into a large, heavy-based saucepan and place over a low–medium heat, then roughly chop the onion and add to the pan. Sauté for about 5 minutes, then slice the mushrooms into quarters and add to the onion. Gently fry for a further 15 minutes, stirring occasionally, until the onion is soft and translucent but not browned.

Pour over the chicken stock, then finely chop the marjoram and add to the mixture with the thyme leaves. Bring the soup to a gentle simmer and leave to cook for 5 minutes. Remove from the heat and allow to cool slightly. Using a hand-held blender or a food processor, blitz the soup until smooth and glossy.

Dice the chicken into 5mm/¼in cubes and add to the soup with the oat cream, stirring in and seasoning with salt and pepper to taste. Warm over a low heat for around 10 minutes or until steaming hot. Chop the parsley, then pour the soup into deep bowls, adding a sprinkling of parsley and a grinding of black pepper.

Butternut Squash and Sweet Potato Soup with Walnut Pesto

Serves 4
Contains nuts
—

1 butternut squash
1 sweet potato
1 fennel bulb
1 large white onion
1 tbsp olive oil
3 cloves of garlic
1.2 litres/2 pints
   vegetable stock
Sea salt and freshly
   ground black pepper

For the pesto
60g/2oz shelled walnuts
Leaves from a large bunch
   of curly-leaf parsley
3 tbsp extra-virgin olive oil
Sea salt and freshly
   ground black pepper

This is a wonderfully velvety soup with an intense flavour, the fennel providing an aromatic contrast to the sweetness of the butternut squash and the walnut pesto lending an earthiness that's just right for an autumnal day. The pesto will make a little more than you need and so is perfect for serving with other things, such as adding to spaghetti or to my White Soda Bread (see page 213). It can be stored in the fridge, covered with a little extra olive oil to preserve it, for up to three days.

Begin by making the pesto. In a heavy-based frying pan, dry-fry the walnuts over a medium–high heat for 6–8 minutes, shaking the pan regularly to ensure they don't burn, until they start to crisp up and you can smell their nutty aroma. Remove from the heat and allow to cool.

Once cool, add the toasted walnuts to a food processor with the parsley, olive oil and a pinch of salt and blitz until you have a coarse paste. Alternatively, pound the ingredients together using a pestle and mortar. Season with pepper and more salt to taste, adding a little more olive oil if necessary, then transfer to a bowl, cover and chill in the fridge until you are ready to use it.

Peel the butternut squash and cut in half, scooping out the seeds and fibres. Peel the sweet potato and trim the fennel, then chop all the vegetables into roughly 2cm/¾in cubes.

Pour the olive oil into a large saucepan set over a low–medium heat, then crush the garlic and add to the pan with the onion and gently sauté for 4–5 minutes or until the onion is soft and translucent but not browned. Add the remaining vegetables and fry with the onion for a further 6–8 minutes or until they soften, starting to give a little when pressed with a wooden spoon.

Season with salt and pepper and pour in the vegetable stock. Cover with a lid and bring to the boil, then reduce the heat and simmer for approximately 25 minutes.

Once the soup is cooked, allow to cool slightly, then, using a hand-held blender or a food processor, blitz until smooth and velvety. Season with salt and pepper to taste, heat through and pour into bowls. Place a heaped teaspoon of the pesto into the middle of each bowl and serve immediately.

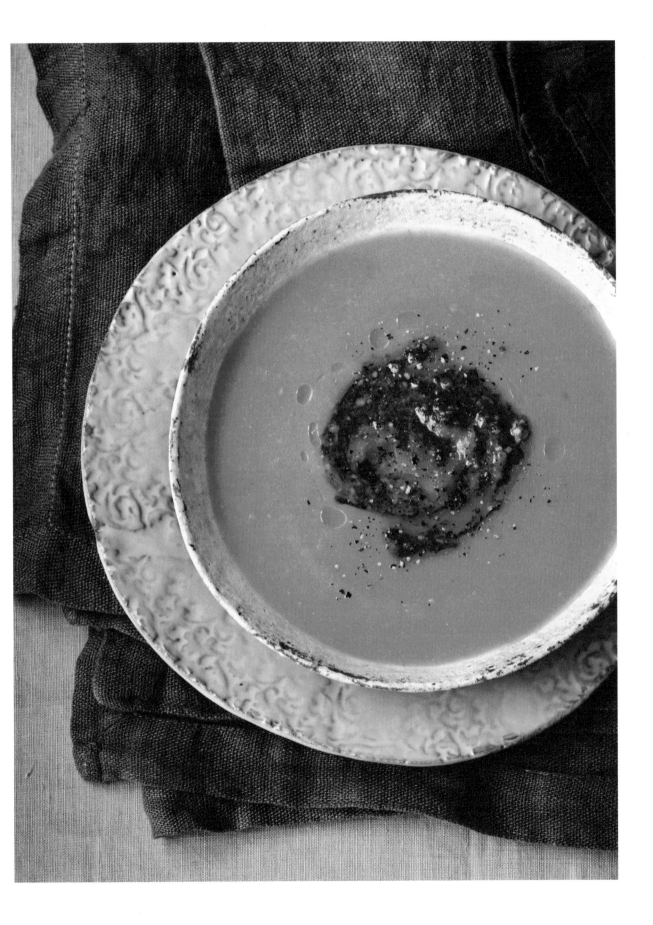

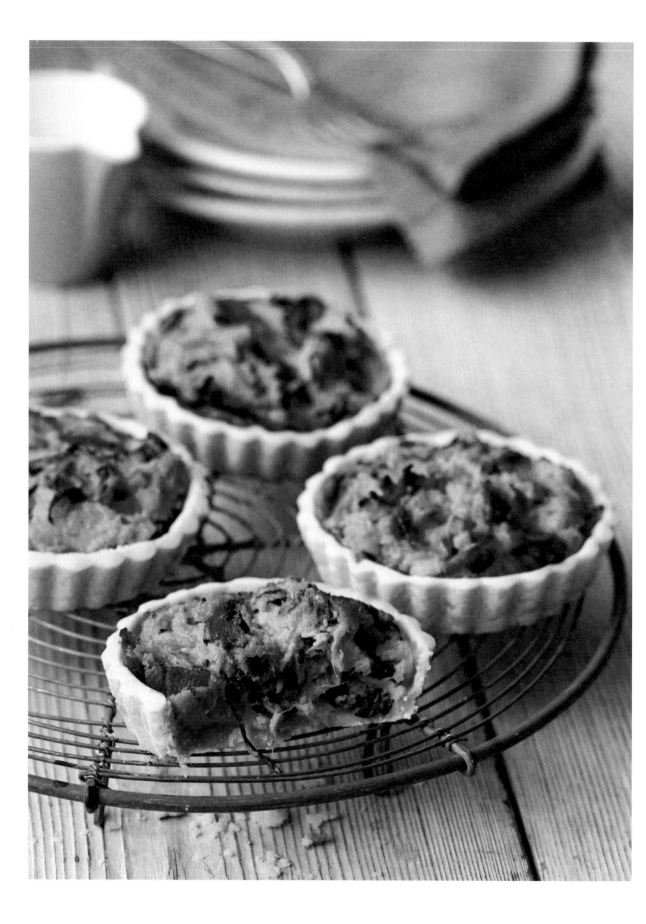

Sweet Potato, Thyme and Bacon Tartlets

**Makes 4 tartlets
or 1 large tart**

—

1 quantity of Shortcrust
Pastry (see page 223)

For the filling
800g/1¾lb sweet
  potatoes
2 cloves of garlic
1 tbsp olive oil
6 rashers of smoked
  streaky bacon
2 handfuls of baby-leaf
  spinach
1 tbsp thyme leaves
Sea salt and freshly
  ground black pepper

*You will need four 11cm/
4½in diameter tart tins
with removable bases (or
one 23cm/9in diameter tart
tin with a removable base)*

Creamy sweet potato combined with crispy smoked bacon and mellow thyme; these little tarts make the ideal starter or light lunch. Serve with a crunchy green salad tossed in a lemon and olive oil dressing.

Begin by making the filling. Peel the sweet potatoes and cut into 5cm/2in chunks, then slice the garlic into thin rounds and set aside for later. Bring a large saucepan of salted water to the boil, add the sweet potato and cook for around 10 minutes or until the potato feels soft to the point of a knife. Drain the sweet potatoes, then tip back into the pan, add the olive oil, season well with salt and pepper and mash vigorously into a smooth purée. (It helps to beat the mixture with a wooden spoon every now and then before continuing to mash.) Set aside to cool down slightly.

In a heavy-based frying pan, dry-fry the bacon rashers on each side over a medium–high heat for around 3 minutes or until crisp, then remove from the pan and set aside. Add the garlic to the pan and fry in the leftover bacon fat for a minute or two then add the spinach leaves, sauté over a low heat for 2–3 minutes or until the spinach has completely wilted. Cut the bacon into small pieces and stir into the puréed sweet potato with the spinach, garlic and thyme, seasoning with salt and pepper to taste.

Preheat the oven to 180°C/350°C/gas mark 4.

Cut the pastry into quarters (for individual tarts; leave whole for a single, large tart), then roll out and fill the tart tins (or single, large tin) following the instructions given in the Shortcrust Pastry recipe on page 223.

Fill each tart to the top with the sweet potato mixture, then place in the oven and cook for 30–35 minutes (40–45 minutes for one large tart) or until the pastry is slightly crisp and the filling just starting to brown on top. Allow to cool slightly, then carefully remove from the tins (or tin) and serve while warm.

Salmon Carpaccio with Caper Dressing

Serves 8

—

800g/1lb very fresh
    salmon fillet, with the
    skin removed (you can
    ask your fishmonger
    to do this for you)
2 lemons
A small bunch of dill
1 red onion
2 tsp caster sugar
1 tsp sea salt
2 tbsp olive oil
1 tbsp capers, drained
    and rinsed

This dish works brilliantly as an effortless no-cook starter or as part of a big spread for a celebratory meal – you could even make it the day ahead for a truly stress-free beginning to your gathering. Equally, it's lovely served as a party nibble – slice up some dense, yeast-free Rye Soda Bread (see page 214) to eat with it and let people help themselves. I recommend a glass of champagne to keep it company!

Begin by rinsing and drying the piece of salmon, then wrap it in cling film and put in the freezer for 1 hour (this will make it easier to slice).

Finely grate the zest of one of the lemons and squeeze the juice from both, passing it through a fine sieve to ensure no pith or pips remain. Finely chop the dill and onion, then add to a bowl with the sugar, salt, olive oil, capers and lemon zest and juice. Whisk all the ingredients together until fully amalgamated.

Unwrap the salmon and, using a very sharp knife, cut off wafer-thin slices, as you would for smoked salmon. Arrange the salmon slices on a large flat dish and spoon over the dressing so that it finds its way into every crease and crevice of the fish. Cover with cling film and chill for at least 2 hours or overnight before serving.

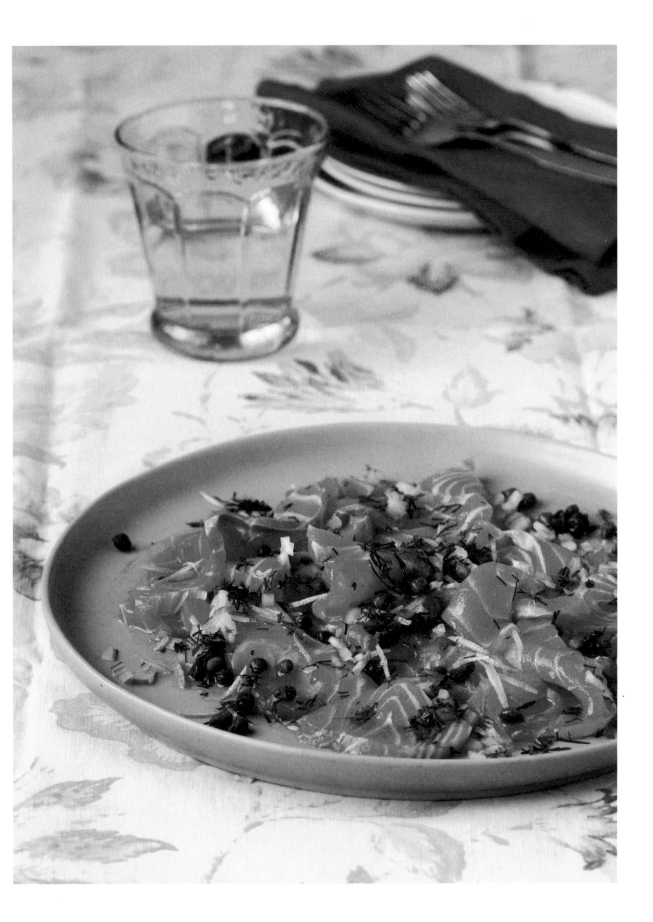

Smoked Chicken, Butternut Squash and Avocado Salad

Serves 4
Contains nuts

—

1 small butternut squash
2 tbsp olive oil
20g/¾oz pine nuts
1 large cos lettuce
12 cherry tomatoes
2 smoked chicken breasts
1 ripe avocado
A small bunch of coriander
Juice of ½ lemon
Sea salt and freshly
  ground black pepper

The balance and contrast of colour and flavour in this salad makes for the most delicious autumnal fare. It has a great combination of taste and texture – the smoky chicken breast mixed with the sweet roasted squash, cool avocado and crunchy toasted pine nuts. Delightful served either as a starter divided between four, or as a satisfying lunch for two.

Preheat the oven to 200°C/400°F/gas mark 6.

First cut the butternut squash lengthways into quarters, leaving the skin on, and scoop out the seeds and fibres. Place on a baking tray, drizzle with half the olive oil and season well with salt and pepper, then roast in the oven for 30 minutes or until tender to the point of a knife.

Meanwhile, scatter the pine nuts on a baking tray and toast in the oven, turning them occasionally to make sure they don't burn, for 5–6 minutes or until golden brown, then remove and set aside to cool.

While the butternut squash is still cooking, shred the lettuce and lay on a large platter or divide between individual plates, to form the base of the salad. Halve the cherry tomatoes and cut the chicken breasts into slices 1cm/½in thick. Cut the avocado in half and remove the stone, then scoop out the flesh and cut into small chunks, scattering these over the lettuce with the tomatoes and slices of chicken.

Finely chop the coriander and set aside, then combine the lemon juice with the remaining olive oil, season well with salt and pepper and whisk together.

When the butternut squash has finished cooking, remove from the oven and allow to cool slightly before handling. Carefully peel away the skin and discard, then cut the flesh into 2cm/¾in chunks and add this to the salad. Pour over the dressing and lightly toss all the ingredients together, then scatter over the chopped coriander and toasted pine nuts to serve.

Chicken and Sweet Potato Casserole

Serves 4

—

1 large white onion
2 sticks of celery
3 cloves of garlic
1 sweet potato
1 tbsp gluten-free plain
  flour (ideally Doves Farm)
8 chicken thighs on the
  bone (skin left on)
2 tbsp olive oil
500ml/18fl oz chicken
  stock
175g/6oz brown
  basmati rice
A small bunch of
  marjoram
2 tbsp English mustard
  (2 tbsp mustard powder
  mixed with 2 tbsp water)
Grated zest of 1 lemon
Sea salt and freshly
  ground black pepper

*You will need a large,
heavy-based casserole dish
with a lid for this recipe*

This dish is a melodic blend of soul foods. The flavours are simple – a little garlic here, some sharp lemon there, a murmur of marjoram, the sugary starch of sweet potato, a burst of heat from the mustard and the pure, restorative taste of chicken stock binding it all together. The beauty of this dish is that it cooks together slowly: the rice soaking up the stock and the chicken braising until it becomes so tender the meat just falls from the bone. If you need a little uplifting, then this dish is the one for you.

Preheat the oven to 180°C/350°F/gas mark 4.

Begin by finely chopping the onion, celery and garlic. Next, peel the sweet potato and cut into rounds about 5mm/¼in thick. Sprinkle the flour over a dinner plate and season well with salt and pepper, then toss the chicken thighs in the flour until lightly coated all over.

Pour the olive oil into the casserole dish set over a medium heat, add the chicken and seal the meat, turning regularly, for around 5 minutes or until a deep golden all over. Remove the chicken from the pan and set aside. Pour the stock into a separate saucepan and bring it to a low simmer.

Next, lower the heat slightly beneath the casserole dish and add the onion, garlic and celery. Fry for 4–5 minutes, stirring regularly, until softened but not browned. Pour in the rice and fry for a further minute or so, until the grains look a little glassy, then chop the marjoram and stir into the rice mixture with the sweet potato, mustard and lemon zest. Pour in the hot chicken stock and return the chicken thighs to the dish.

Season with salt and pepper, cover the casserole dish tightly with its lid and bring to the boil. Place in the oven and bake for 45–50 minutes or until the rice has soaked up all the stock and the chicken is completely tender. Serve from the casserole dish while hot.

Lebanese Chicken

Serves 4–6

—

900g/2lb floury potatoes
  (ideally Maris Piper)
3–5 lemons
16 cloves of garlic
150ml/5fl oz olive oil
1½ tsp soft light brown
  sugar
3 tbsp egg- and soya-free
  mayonnaise
1 tsp harissa paste
1 tbsp tomato purée
3 boneless chicken breasts
  and 4 chicken thighs on
  the bone (skin left on)
1 x 400g tin of chickpeas,
  drained and rinsed
A small bunch of coriander
A small bunch of mint
Sea salt and freshly
  ground black pepper

*You will need a tagine or
a shallow, heavy-based
casserole dish with a
lid for this recipe*

This dish has the wonderfully pungent flavour of the Middle East and is much loved by family and friends, who are forever asking for the recipe. I would recommend that you marinate the chicken overnight or at the very least for a few hours; it makes all the difference to the flavour. I know that it may seem like a lot of lemon and garlic, but trust me – the result is a triumph. The smell alone will imbue your home with the most delectable tang. You'll need either three large lemons or five smaller ones and try to use Maris Piper potatoes if you can; they seem to be the best at absorbing the juices while still becoming golden and crisp. See my Butternut Squash Tagine (page 148) for a simple harissa recipe. Alternatively, you can buy ready-mixed harissa in supermarkets or specialist stores. Serve with steamed white basmati rice and a large green salad.

Peel and cut the potatoes into 4cm/1½in chunks. Squeeze the juice from the lemons, passing it through a fine sieve to ensure no pith or pips remain. Peel all the garlic cloves and crush eight of them, leaving the remaining ones whole.

Pour the lemon juice and olive oil into a large bowl, add the sugar, mayonnaise, harissa paste and tomato purée and whisk together until thick and creamy. Add the chicken, potatoes, chickpeas and garlic, season with salt and pepper and stir together thoroughly, making sure that all the ingredients are well coated in the marinade. Cover and leave to marinate in the fridge for between 3 and 24 hours, removing it from the fridge an hour or so before cooking to bring it back up to room temperature.

Shortly before you are ready to cook, preheat the oven to 200°C/400°F/gas mark 6.

Transfer the chicken, potatoes and chickpeas to the tagine or casserole dish and pour in the remaining marinade, then cover with the lid and cook in the oven for 1 hour. Take the dish from the oven and remove the lid, then return to the oven and cook for a further 40–45 minutes or until the chicken and potatoes are crisp, golden and bubbling. Finely chop the coriander and mint and sprinkle this over the dish to serve.

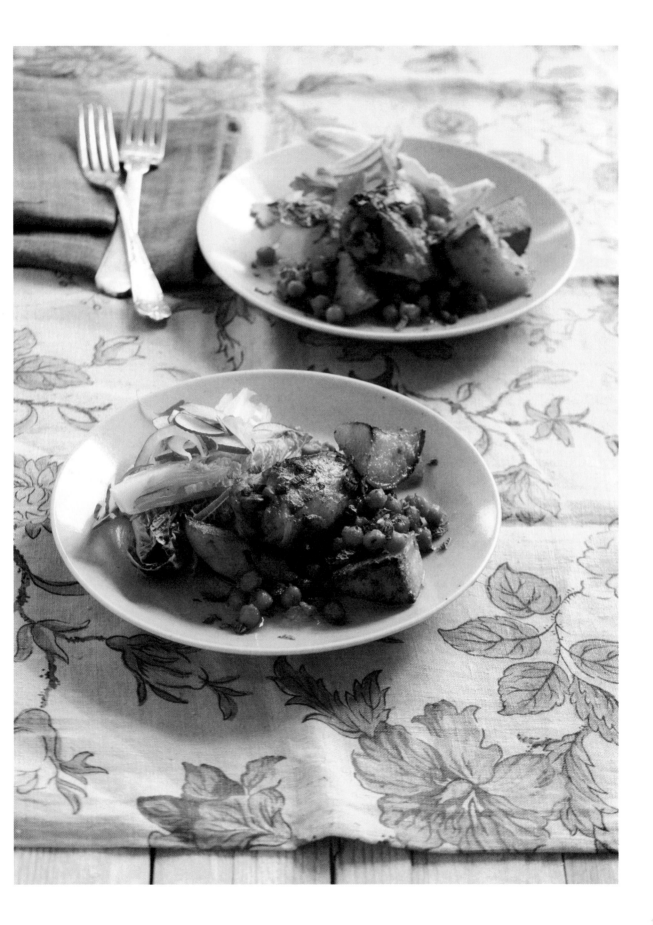

Slow-cooked Spanish Chicken with Chorizo

Serves 4

—

1 tbsp dairy-free margarine (ideally Pure Sunflower Spread)

1 tsp saffron threads

1 tbsp soft light brown sugar

1 tbsp smoked paprika

4 boneless chicken breasts and 4 chicken thighs on the bone (skin left on)

1 tbsp lemon juice

8 cloves of garlic

300g/11oz cooking chorizo

1 tbsp olive oil

2 x 400g tin of chopped tomatoes

2 x 400g tin of butterbeans, drained and rinsed

A bunch of flat-leaf parsley

Sea salt and freshly ground black pepper

You will need a large, heavy-based casserole dish with a lid for this recipe

Whenever I cook with paprika, garlic and saffron, I think of Spain and all its fabulous, fragrant dishes. Here, the slow-baking of the chicken produces melt-in-the-mouth meat that simply falls off the bone. The garlic cloves become sweet and gooey, their mellow flavour melding with the smoky kick of the paprika and the spiciness of the chorizo, while the butterbeans provide a warm base note as well as absorbing all the wonderful juices from the meat. This recipe is ideal for a relaxed supper with friends – just set the dish on the table with a big bowl of steaming basmati rice and a herby green salad tossed in lemon juice and olive oil. Or for a quick and simple meal, serve with chunks of bread to soak up the delicious juices.

Preheat the oven to 150°C/300°F/gas mark 2.

Place the margarine in a bowl with the saffron, sugar and paprika and beat together until creamy, seasoning well with salt and pepper. Cut the chicken breasts in half lengthways and then rub the saffron butter into the skin of all the chicken pieces. Pour over the lemon juice and set aside while you peel the garlic cloves (leaving them whole) and cut the chorizo into half-moons.

Pour the olive oil into the casserole dish and fry the chorizo over a medium–high heat for 3–4 minutes or until it begins to turn crisp and release its paprika-spiked oils.

Remove the dish from the heat and add the tomatoes, garlic and butterbeans to the chorizo, and mix together, seasoning lightly with salt and pepper. Place the chicken, skin side up, on top of the beans, cover with a lid and bake in the oven for 2¼ hours.

Remove from the oven, take off the lid and increase the oven temperature to 200°C/400°F/gas mark 6. Return the dish to the oven and continue to bake for a further 15 minutes or until the chicken is crisp and golden. Finely chop the parsley and sprinkle over the chicken to serve.

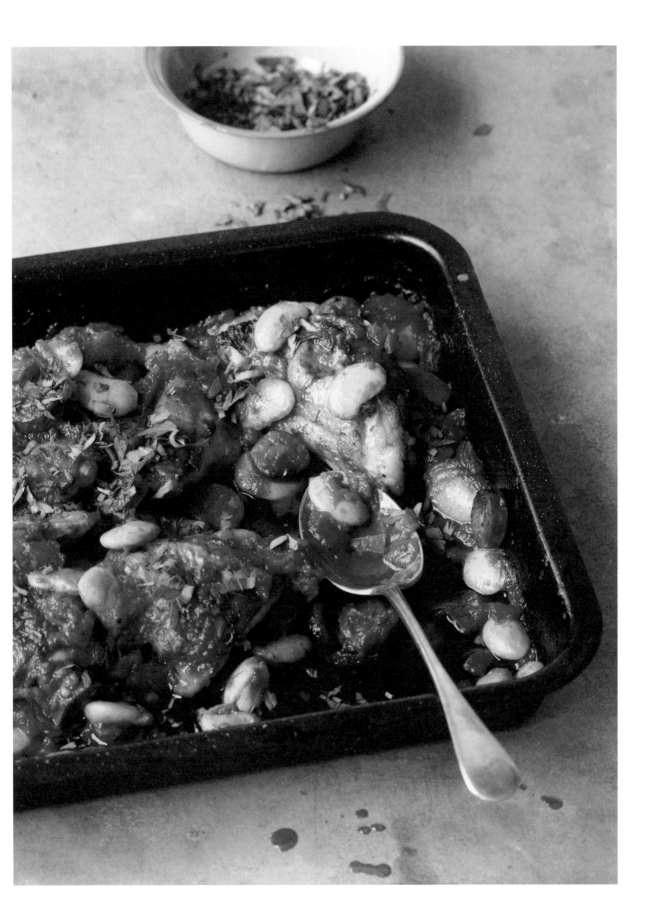

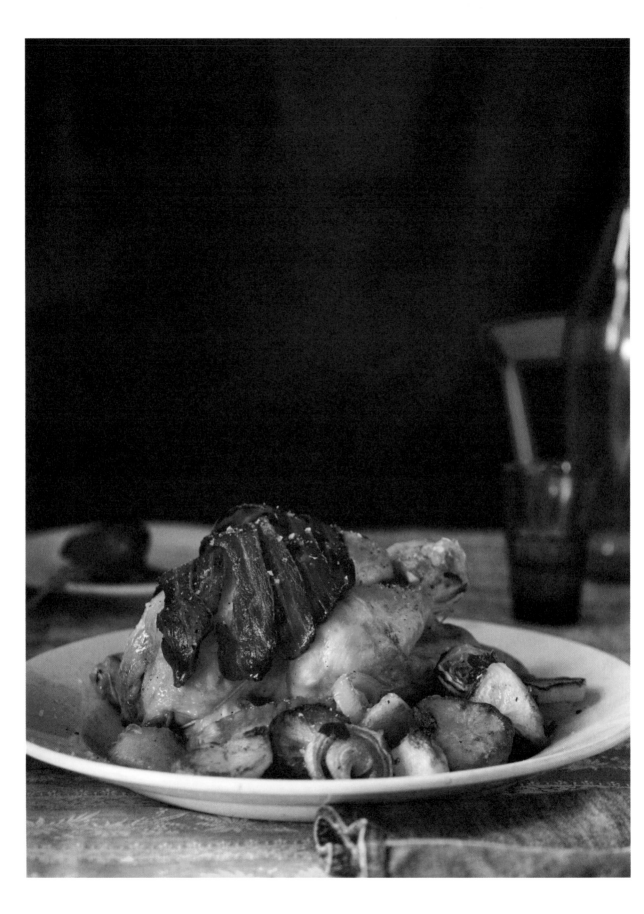

Roast Chicken with Sage and Garlic and Perfect Roast Potatoes

Serves 4

—

2 large white onions
A small bunch of sage
4 cloves of garlic (unpeeled)
1 tbsp lemon juice
1 tbsp soft light brown
　sugar
150ml/5fl oz chicken
　stock or water
1 x 1.6kg/3½lb chicken
6 rashers of smoked
　streaky bacon
Sea salt and freshly
　ground black pepper

For the roast potatoes
8 floury potatoes
　(such as Maris Piper
　or Lady Balfour)
4 tbsp groundnut or
　rapeseed oil
1 heaped tsp sea salt

For the gravy
300ml/½ pint hot
　chicken stock
1½ tbsp cornflour

For the English, the Sunday roast is a national institution and autumn is the perfect time to start partaking of this delicious tradition. I know it's contentious, but I like to cook the chicken and the roast potatoes separately, to ensure the potatoes remain as crisp as possible and aren't the least bit soggy. I also like to roast my chicken on a layer of onions, which soften in a delicious creamy pile during cooking. For maximum pleasure, serve to your family and friends with a big bowl of seasonal vegetables.

Preheat the oven to 240°C/475°F/gas mark 9 and ensure that there are two shelves ready – one at the bottom of the oven for the chicken and the other near the top for the potatoes.

Slice the onions into rounds about 1cm/½in thick and roughly chop the sage, then place both in a large roasting tin or ovenproof dish with the garlic, lemon juice, sugar and chicken stock or water. Season well with salt and pepper and mix together. Rest the chicken on top of the onions, lay the bacon rashers over the chicken and season with more salt and pepper.

Place in the oven and immediately reduce the temperature to 220°C/425°F/gas mark 7. Roast for 1 hour and 10 minutes or until the chicken is golden and, when pierced with a skewer, the juices run clear. (Always test the meat of the thigh rather than the breast as it is the slowest to cook.) Remove the chicken from the oven, then carefully lift it out of the tin, setting the tin with the cooking juices to one side, and place on a large platter or serving plate. Using a slotted spoon, scoop out the roasted onions and place underneath the chicken. Cover the chicken with foil and allow to rest for at least 10 minutes before carving.

While the chicken is cooking, peel the potatoes and cut into 5cm/2in chunks (roughly 'two bites' worth' in size). Place in a large saucepan of salted water and bring to the boil. The second the water begins to boil, time the potatoes, allowing them to cook for precisely 4 minutes before removing from the heat and draining. Once drained, shake the potatoes in the colander a little so that their edges mar and become rough – this allows the potatoes to become truly crisp and crunchy when roasted. Pour the groundnut or rapeseed oil into a large roasting tin and tip in the potatoes, then sprinkle with the sea salt and firmly shake to coat evenly.

After the chicken has been cooking for 30 minutes, place the potatoes in the oven and roast for the remaining cooking and resting time (40–50 minutes) or until crisp and golden.

recipe continues >

> *continued from*
previous page

Meanwhile, make the gravy. Place the roasting tin with the juices from the roast chicken over a medium heat. Pour in the hot chicken stock, stirring in with a wooden spoon and scraping the bottom of the tin to incorporate all the caramelised bits from the cooked chicken and onions. In a separate bowl, mix the cornflour with 1½ tablespoons of water until smooth, then stir this mixture into the hot stock and simmer gently, stirring continuously, until you have the desired consistency for your gravy.

Remove the potatoes from the oven and serve with the carved chicken, a pile of the softened onions, some pieces of crispy bacon and a spoonful or two of gravy.

Thyme and Chilli Chicken on Pea Purée

Serves 4
—
2 tbsp dairy-free margarine (ideally Pure Sunflower Spread)
1 tbsp chilli powder
¼ tsp ground mace
Leaves from a small bunch of thyme
8 chicken thighs on the bone (skin left on)
Sea salt and freshly ground black pepper

For the pea purée
450g/1lb frozen peas
40ml/1½fl oz oat cream
A few mint leaves
Sea salt and freshly ground black pepper

I love the combination of flavours here: the hot chilli, mellow mace and aromatic thyme mixed into a delicious spiced butter, the finished dish offset by the creamy sweetness of the pea purée. Colourful and fresh yet comforting, this is a lovely dish to make for an autumnal lunch or supper; I would serve it with a few sautéed or boiled potatoes.

Preheat the oven to 220°C/425°F/gas mark 7.

Place the margarine in a bowl with the chilli, mace and thyme leaves and beat together until smooth and creamy. Using a sharp knife and cutting to a depth of about 1cm/½in, score the top of each chicken thigh diagonally 3–4 times and then rub in the spiced butter, pushing it into the gaps and spreading it all over the skin.

Place the chicken, skin side up, in a roasting tin, season well with salt and pepper and then roast in the oven for 40–45 minutes or until the skin is crisp and the meat is tender and, when pierced with a skewer, the juices run clear.

Meanwhile, place the peas in a bowl, cover with boiling water and leave to stand for around 4 minutes. Drain the peas and transfer to a blender, add the oat cream and mint leaves and season well with salt and pepper before blitzing until smooth and thick. Season further to taste, then transfer the purée to a small saucepan and heat gently until ready to serve.

Remove the chicken from the oven, cover in foil and set aside to rest for 5 minutes. Divide the pea purée between warmed plates, spooning it into the centre of each plate and laying two chicken thighs on top.

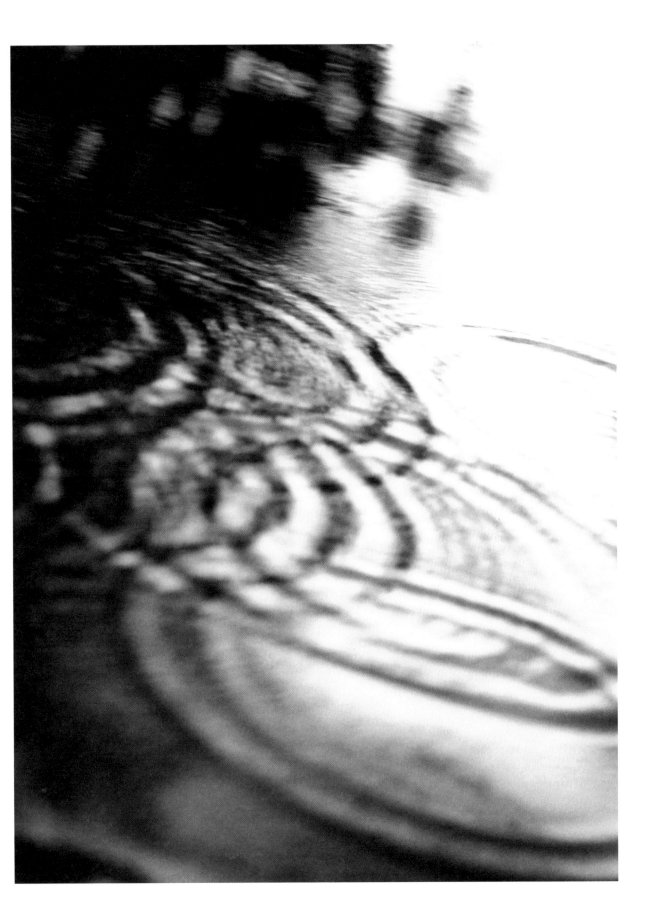

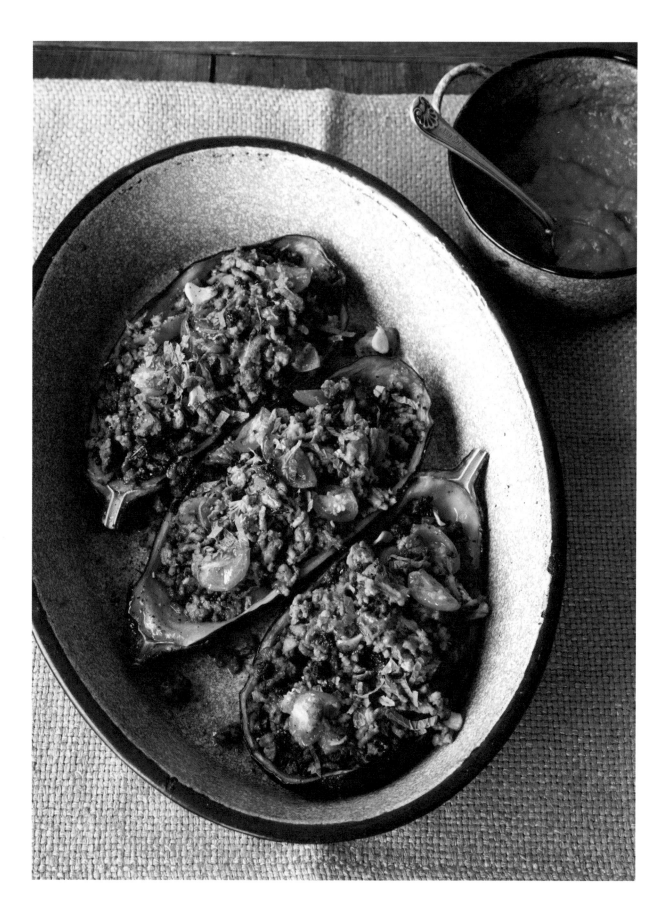

Lamb-stuffed Aubergines with Spiced Tomato Sauce

Serves 4

—

2 large aubergines
1 red onion
12 cherry tomatoes
2 cloves of garlic
A small bunch of mint
2 tbsp olive oil
250g/9oz lean minced
   lamb
1 tsp turmeric
1 tsp ground coriander
Sea salt and freshly
   ground black pepper

*For the spiced
tomato sauce*
1 small red onion
1 small red chilli
1 tbsp olive oil
A pinch of ground cumin
2 tsp soft light brown sugar
1 x 400g tin of chopped
   tomatoes
2 tsp lemon juice
1 tbsp tomato purée
Sea salt and freshly
   ground black pepper

Lamb and aubergine always work well together and this dish has a gloriously intense and earthy depth of flavour. I like to serve it with my Sweet Potato Crouton Rice or my Potatoes with Parsley, Capers and Lemon (see pages 150 and 104) and a herby leaf salad. The sauce is so simple to make and will keep, covered, for up to three days in the fridge.

Begin by making the spiced tomato sauce. Roughly chop the onion, deseed the chilli and finely slice. Heat the olive oil in a frying pan, add the onion, chilli and cumin and fry over a low heat, stirring occasionally, for 10–15 minutes or until completely soft but not browned.

Add the sugar and continue to fry, over a low heat, for 2 minutes. Add the chopped tomatoes, lemon juice and tomato purée to the pan. Cover with a lid, then bring to the boil, reduce the heat to low and leave to simmer for 15 minutes. Allow to cool slightly, then season with salt and pepper and, using a food processor or hand-held blender, blitz until smooth. Set aside while you prepare the aubergines.

Cut the aubergines in half lengthways and scoop out the flesh, being careful not to pierce the skin. Using a food processor or a sharp knife, finely chop the aubergine flesh so that it becomes almost pulpy. Finely dice the onion and cut the tomatoes into quarters, then thinly slice the garlic and finely chop the mint.

Pour half the olive oil into a large, heavy-based frying pan and sauté the onion over a low heat for 5 minutes. Add the aubergine flesh and minced lamb to the pan, season heavily with salt and pepper and continue to fry gently for about 15 minutes or until both the lamb and aubergine are cooked through. Stir in the turmeric and coriander and continue to cook over a low heat for a further 2 minutes.

Preheat the oven to 200°C/400°F/gas mark 6.

Stir the tomatoes and half the mint into the lamb and aubergine. Rub the remaining olive oil into the aubergine skins and then fill with the lamb mixture. Place in a roasting tin and top each aubergine half with the garlic slices, then cover loosely with foil and cook in the oven for 40 minutes.

Meanwhile, heat up the tomato sauce in a small saucepan. Remove the aubergines from the oven, scatter with the remaining mint and serve with the tomato sauce, either drizzled over or in individual pots.

Lamb Tagine with Dates and Peppers

Serves 4–6
Contains nuts
—
30g/1¼oz pine nuts
1kg/2lb 3oz diced lamb
2 red onions
2 red peppers
100g/3½oz pitted dates
3 tbsp olive oil
1 tbsp dairy-free margarine
  (ideally Pure Sunflower
  Spread)
2 tsp turmeric
2 tsp ground cinnamon
1 tsp ground ginger
200ml/7fl oz lamb stock
  or water
1 tbsp runny honey
A small bunch of coriander
A small bunch of mint
Sea salt and freshly
  ground black pepper

*You will need a tagine or
heavy-based casserole dish
with a lid for this recipe*

Rich and fragrant, this tagine is truly heart-warming on a chilly autumn evening. I love the Middle Eastern way of slow-cooking meats until they are dulcet and tender. Equally so their love of merging sweet and spicy flavours and use of ingredients that really lend themselves to intolerance-friendly cooking. You could serve this tagine with some white basmati rice and perhaps a few fresh green leaves for a simple supper. Or you could make a true feast to share with family and friends by including my Flatbreads (see page 221), drizzled with olive oil and sprinkled with sea salt, the Stuffed Aubergines with Sweet Potato Crouton Rice (see page 150) and a bowl of houmous. If you have a proper terracotta tagine, then do use it for this recipe; otherwise, a heavy-based casserole dish will do just as well.

In a heavy based frying pan, dry-fry the pine nuts over a medium heat for 3–4 minutes or until golden brown, shaking the pan regularly to ensure that they don't burn. Remove from the heat and allow to cool.

Trim any obvious excess fat from the pieces of lamb, finely dice the onions and deseed the peppers before slicing them lengthways into thin strips. Cut the dates into pieces approximately 2cm/¾in thick.

Heat the oil and the margarine in the tagine or casserole dish and, when the margarine has melted, fry the onion over a medium heat for 5–6 minutes or until soft and beginning to turn golden. Stir in the spices and fry for a further minute or so, then add the lamb and fry for another minute, stirring it well to ensure that all the meat is well coated in the spices.

Pour over the stock or water and season with salt and pepper. Cover with the lid and bring to the boil, then reduce the heat to its lowest setting and simmer very gently for 1½ hours. Alternatively, place in the oven, preheated to 160°C/325°F/gas mark 3, and cook for the same length of time.

Stir in the dates, honey and sliced red pepper, then cover again and continue to simmer gently (or return to the oven) for a further 30 minutes or until the meat is tender and falling apart. Meanwhile, finely chop the coriander and mint. Remove the tagine or casserole dish from the hob or oven and scatter over the chopped herbs and toasted pine nuts to serve.

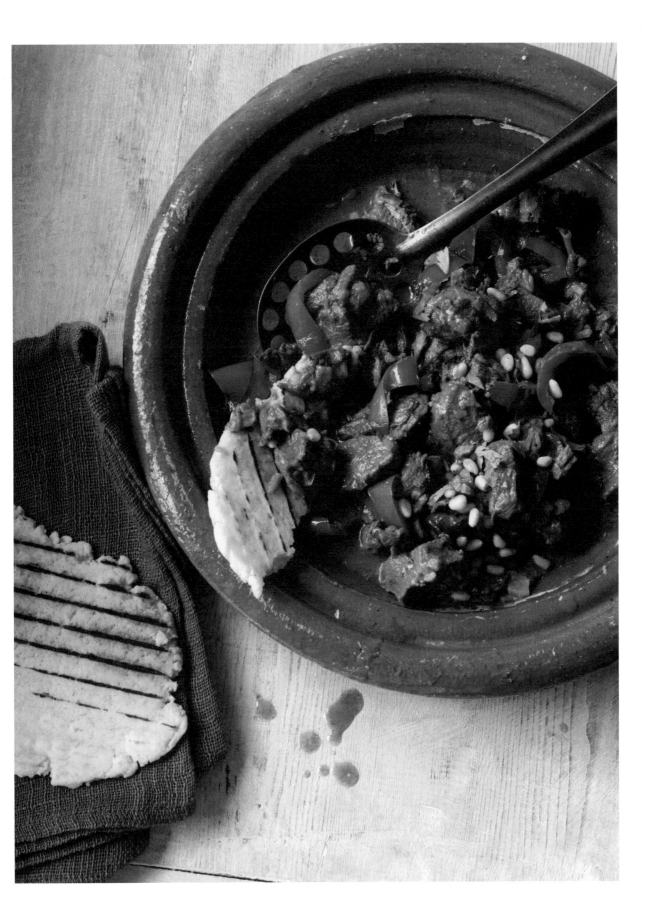

Spaghetti Carbonara

Serves 4
Contains nuts
—

50g/1¾oz pine nuts
150ml/5fl oz oat cream
175g/6oz smoked pancetta
2 fat cloves of garlic
A small bunch of flat-leaf
   parsley
1 tbsp olive oil
350g/12oz gluten-free
   spaghetti
Sea salt and freshly
   ground black pepper

Spaghetti carbonara, with its rich sauce of egg yolks and cheese, may not be the first dish you'd expect to find in an intolerance-friendly cookbook. To try to reproduce this medley of textures and flavours for a dairy-, egg- and gluten-free version of the recipe, I've used a combination of pine nuts, toasted and ground, and oat cream to recreate the depth and bite that you would get from mixing egg yolks and Parmesan cheese. I've included pancetta, as in the original dish, plus a scattering of parsley to add a fresh note. This is a real winner for autumn and will have you feeling cosy and warm before you've even taken your first mouthful.

In a heavy-based frying pan, dry-fry the pine nuts over a medium–high heat for 3–4 minutes or until golden brown, shaking the pan regularly to ensure that they don't burn. Remove from the heat and allow to cool slightly. Once cool enough to handle, use a food processor or pestle and mortar to grind them to the consistency of fine breadcrumbs.

Mix the ground pine nuts and oat cream together in a bowl, add ½ teaspoon of salt and whisk together until you have a rich and smooth sauce.

Cut the pancetta into 5mm/¼in cubes, crush the garlic and finely chop the parsley. Pour the olive oil into the heavy-based frying pan and place over a medium–high heat, then add the pancetta and garlic and sauté for 4–5 minutes or until golden and crispy.

Meanwhile, bring a large saucepan of salted water to the boil, add the spaghetti and cook until al dente following the instructions on the packet – usually 10–12 minutes, depending on the brand of pasta. While the spaghetti is cooking, pour the cream sauce over the fried pancetta and mix thoroughly, then heat through gently so that the sauce becomes hot but without boiling.

Once the spaghetti is cooked, drain and then return to the pan, pour over the carbonara sauce and combine gently, ensuring that the spaghetti is entirely coated in the sauce. Serve hot, sprinkled with the chopped parsley and with a little freshly ground pepper.

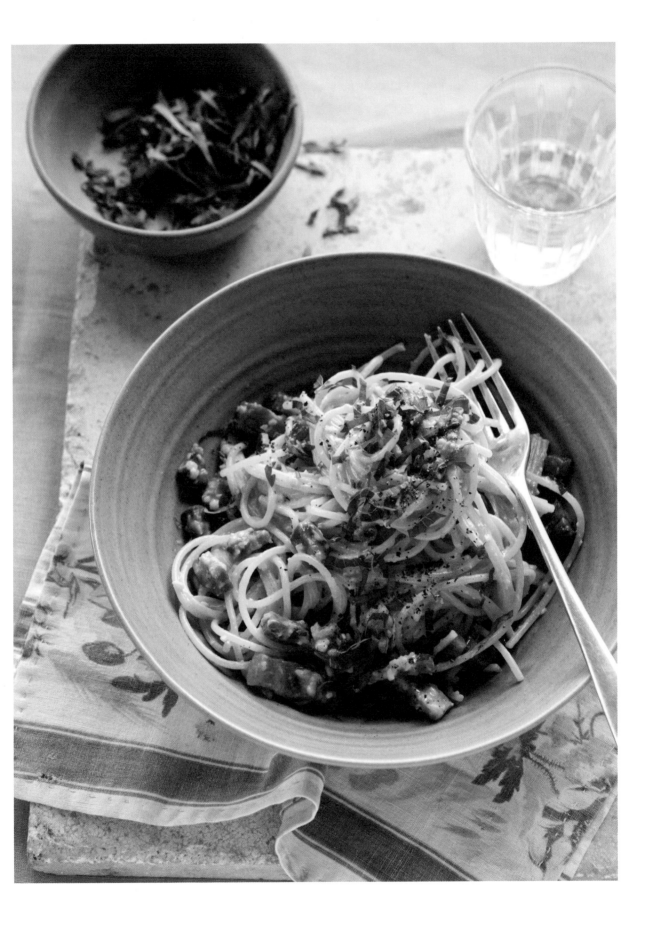

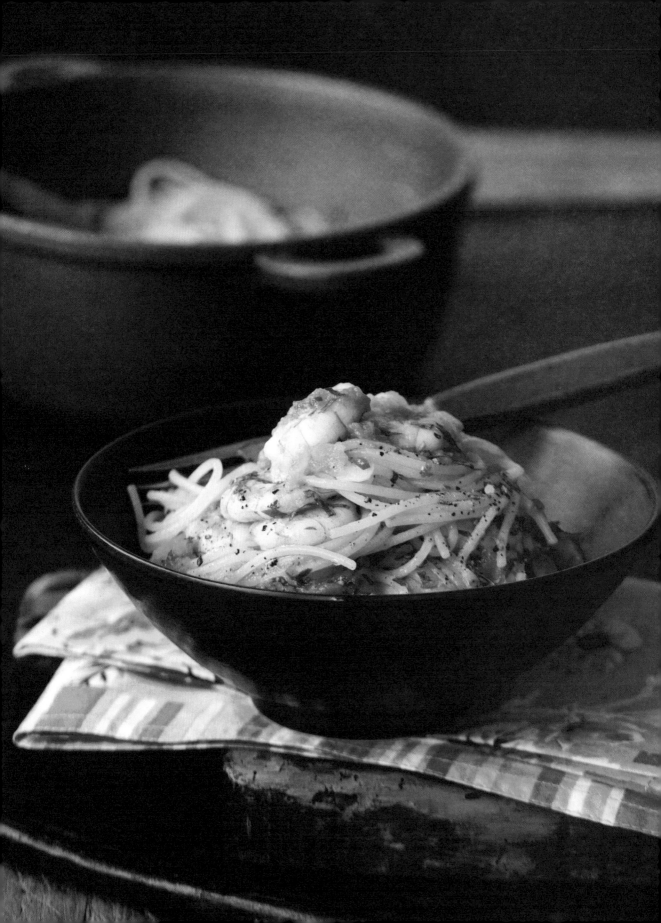

Prawn Arrabbiata

Serves 4

—

1kg/2lb 3oz ripe plum
 tomatoes or vine-
 ripened tomatoes
350g/12oz gluten-free
 spaghetti
½ red chilli
4 cloves of garlic
3 tbsp olive oil
1 tsp lemon juice
1 tsp soft light brown
 sugar
A small bunch of basil
A small bunch of
 curly-leaf parsley
250g/9oz cooked and
 peeled tiger prawns
Sea salt and freshly
 ground black pepper

*Despite its name – arrabbiata means 'angry-style' in Italian, for the heat
of the chilli – this dish has a very clean taste and leaves you feeling both
nourished and indulged. Using fresh tomatoes makes all the difference,
their tangy flavour complementing the kick of the chilli and mild
sweetness of the prawns. Ideally you want to use ripe plum tomatoes,
but vine-ripened tomatoes would do equally well. Don't be tempted to
omit the lemon juice and brown sugar; both are essential for enhancing
the flavour of the tomatoes.*

First skin the tomatoes by placing them in a large bowl, covering with
boiling water and leaving for 1 minute. Drain and then carefully peel
away the tomato skins (they should slide off with ease), slice in half
and scoop out the seeds. Roughly chop the flesh and set aside.

Meanwhile, bring a large saucepan of lightly salted water to the boil,
add the pasta and cook until al dente following the instructions on the
packet – usually 10–12 minutes, depending on the brand. While the
pasta is cooking, finely chop the chilli, retaining the seeds, and finely
slice the garlic into rounds.

Pour the olive oil into another large saucepan, over a low–medium
heat, add the garlic and chilli and a good pinch of salt (to stop the garlic
burning) and sauté gently until softened. Add the tomatoes to the pan,
along with the lemon juice and brown sugar, then raise the heat to
medium–high and cook for 5 minutes or until the tomatoes have
broken down, forming a loose sauce.

Roughly chop the basil and parsley and add to the pan with the
prawns, season well with salt and pepper and continue to cook for
another minute or so. Drain the pasta and add it to the sauce. Stir all
the ingredients together so that the pasta moves fluidly in the sauce,
then season further to taste and serve immediately.

Peppers Stuffed with Chestnuts, Chilli and Butternut Squash

Serves 4
Contains nuts

—

1 butternut squash
2 tbsp olive oil
4 red peppers
1 red onion
12 cherry tomatoes
200g/7oz cooked and
   peeled chestnuts
Leaves from a small
   bunch of thyme
½ tsp chilli flakes
Sea salt and freshly
   ground black pepper

Bursting with flavour, texture and colour, this is such a satisfying dish. The sweet but meaty quality of the chestnuts, creaminess of the butternut squash and the hint of chilli combine together in a way that is truly pleasing to the palate. I like to serve this with some white basmati rice and perhaps a little kale sautéed in garlic and olive oil or on a bed of rocket with a few potato wedges. If you want to make extra, these peppers are delicious served cold the next day, scattered with some toasted pine nuts. They also freeze very well and can be cooked in the oven from frozen at around 150°C/300°F/gas mark 2 for an hour – but do cover them again in foil before popping in the oven.

Preheat the oven to 200°C/400°F/gas mark 6.

Slice the butternut squash lengthways into quarters, leaving the skin on, then scoop out the seeds and fibres and discard. Place on a baking tray and drizzle each quarter with half the olive oil, then season with salt and pepper and bake in the oven for 45 minutes or until cooked through and tender. Remove from the oven and allow to cool.

Cut each red pepper in half lengthways, slicing through the stalk so that each half has part of its stalk left attached. Carefully remove the seeds and white pith from each pepper, cutting around the stalk, then halve the onion and slice into thin half-moons. Pour the remaining olive oil into a saucepan and gently sauté the onion over a low heat for 10 minutes or until completely soft but not browned.

Using a sharp knife, cut away the skin from the cooked butternut squash, then cut the flesh into small chunks and add to the onion. Slice the cherry tomatoes and chestnuts in half and add to the pan with the thyme leaves. Sprinkle over the chilli flakes, season with salt and pepper and mix together.

Lay each red pepper half on a baking tray and carefully fill with the squash and chestnut mixture. Cover loosely with foil and bake in the oven for 50 minutes and serve while hot.

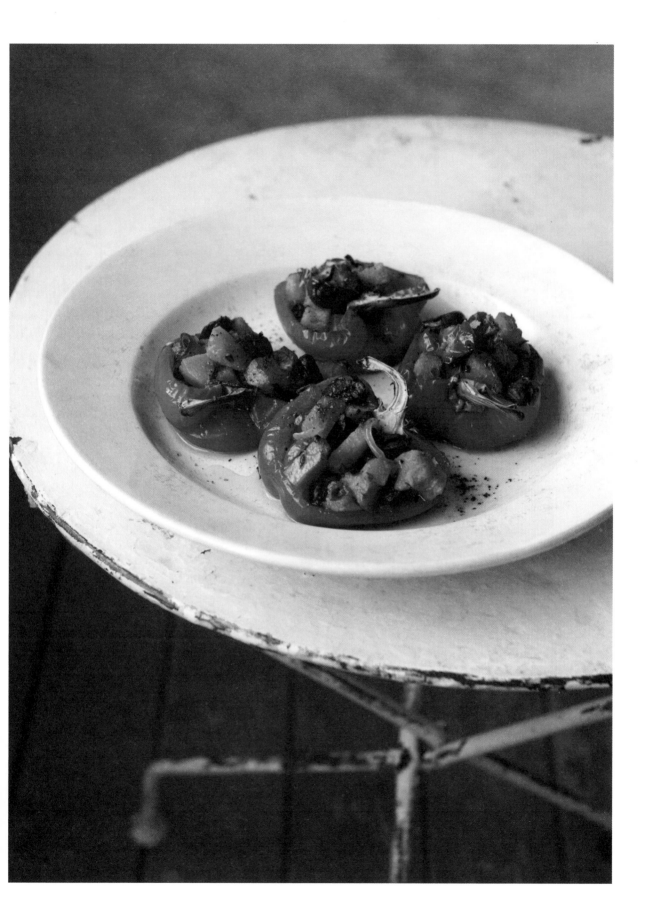

Butternut Squash Tagine

Serves 4
Contains nuts
—

1 large butternut squash
2 large red onions
8 cloves of garlic
3 tbsp olive oil
1 tsp dairy-free margarine
(ideally Pure Sunflower
Spread)
125g/4½oz sultanas
2 tbsp agave syrup or
runny honey
1 x 400g tin of chickpeas,
drained and rinsed
75g/3oz flaked almonds
A small bunch of coriander
Sea salt and freshly
ground black pepper

For the harissa paste
2 cloves of garlic
½ tsp sea salt
4 tsp chilli flakes
(smoked if possible)
1 tsp ground coriander
1 tsp ground cumin
¼ tsp ground cinnamon
4 tbsp olive oil

*You will need a tagine or
heavy-based casserole dish
with a lid for this recipe*

This tagine is gloriously warming with a melodious sweet note and golden hues fitting for the season. You could serve it as it is, with a big bowl of basmati rice to soak up those lovely juices. It also goes well with Flatbreads (see page 221), houmous and a large herb salad. If you don't feel like making your own harissa, then you can easily buy it in a supermarket or specialist shop. The harissa recipe here will make more than you need for this dish. To store, simply transfer to a small jar or plastic container, cover with a thin layer of olive oil and a lid and keep in the fridge. Kept this way, it will last for up to ten days and is ideal for stirring into sauces or using as a marinade.

First prepare the harissa. Roughly chop the garlic and, using a pestle and mortar, pound this with the salt, chilli flakes and spices until you have a thick paste, then stir in the olive oil, bit by bit, to bind the paste together.

Next, cut the butternut squash in half lengthways, scoop out the seeds and fibres and cut away the peel, then slice widthways into strips about 2.5cm/1in wide. Slice the onions into quarters and flatten the garlic cloves with a wooden spatula so that they become lightly crushed and their juices start to leak out.

Heat the oil and margarine in the tagine or casserole dish and, when the margarine has melted, stir in the onions and garlic and sauté them over a medium–high heat for about 5 minutes or until they begin to brown. Add the sultanas, agave syrup or honey and 2 teaspoons of the harissa paste and stir into the onions. Add the butternut squash and chickpeas to the dish and carefully mix so that everything is well coated in the rich, spicy harissa.

Pour in 50–75ml/2–3fl oz water (enough to cover the base of the dish), then season with salt and pepper and cover with the lid. Cook over a low heat for 25–30 minutes or until the onions and squash are tender to the point of a knife but still hold their shape. Alternatively, place the dish in the oven, preheated to 180°C/350°F/gas mark 4, and cook for the same length of time.

In a heavy-based frying pan, dry-fry the flaked almonds over a medium–high heat for 1–2 minutes or until golden brown in colour, shaking the pan regularly to ensure that they don't burn, and then leave to cool for a minute while you finely chop the coriander. Serve the tagine sprinkled with the toasted almonds and chopped coriander.

Spaghetti with Roasted Aubergine, Thyme and Chilli Sauce

Serves 4
Contains nuts
—

2 aubergines
Leaves from 8 sprigs
of thyme
6 tbsp olive oil
30g/1¼oz pine nuts
1 red onion
2 cloves of garlic
1 large mild red chilli
or 1 tsp chilli flakes
(smoked if possible)
1 heaped tsp soft light
brown sugar
2 tsp tomato purée
2 tsp lemon juice
A handful of pitted
black olives
1 x 400g tin of chopped
tomatoes
350g/12oz gluten-free
spaghetti
Sea salt and freshly
ground black pepper

This sauce is inspired by the Mediterranean flavours of ratatouille and Sicilian caponata (an aubergine dish). The aubergine is baked until its flesh is tender and crisp, permeated with the warming fragrance of thyme, chilli and garlic. The black olives lend a salty kick while the pine nuts bolster the sauce with body and bite. You can replace the sprigs of thyme with a handful of capers, but I cannot champion the pairing of thyme and aubergine enough – the combination of creamy, dusky aubergine with aromatic thyme is, in my view, a match made in heaven.

Preheat the oven to 200°C/400°F/gas mark 6.

Cut the aubergines into 1cm/½in cubes and combine with the thyme leaves in a roasting tin. Add 4 tablespoons of the olive oil and mix thoroughly so that the aubergines are well coated in the oil, then roast in the oven for 40 minutes or until softened and starting to crisp on top. (The aubergine may be a little charred at the edges, but this is fine – it'll just add to the flavour.)

While the aubergines are cooking, scatter the pine nuts on a baking tray and toast in the oven, turning them occasionally to make sure they don't burn, for 5–6 minutes or until golden brown, then remove and set aside to cool.

Meanwhile, finely dice the onion and crush the garlic. If using the fresh chilli, deseed it and then finely dice. Heat the remaining olive oil in a large, heavy-based saucepan and sauté the onions, garlic and fresh chilli (if using) over a low–medium heat for 10 minutes or until soft and translucent but not browned. Add the chilli flakes (if using), sugar, tomato purée and lemon juice to the onions, season well with salt and pepper and sauté gently for a further minute or two.

Finely slice the black olives into rounds and add them to the onion mixture. Pour over the tomatoes and stir in, then cover with a lid and bring to the boil. Once boiling, reduce the heat and leave to simmer over a very low heat for 20 minutes. Once the aubergine is cooked, remove from the oven, season well with salt and pepper and add to the sauce. Cover again and continue to cook over a low heat for a further 10 minutes.

Meanwhile, bring a large saucepan of salted water to the boil, add the spaghetti and cook until al dente following the instructions on the packet – usually 10–12 minutes, depending on the brand of pasta. Once cooked, drain and drizzle with olive oil and season with sea salt. Add the spaghetti to the aubergine and tomato sauce, gently combining until the spaghetti is glossy and well coated. Serve sprinkled with the toasted pine nuts.

Stuffed Aubergines with Sweet Potato Crouton Rice

Serves 4

—

2 large aubergines
1 red onion
12 cherry tomatoes
2 cloves of garlic
A small bunch of mint
2 tbsp olive oil
1 tsp turmeric
1 tsp ground coriander
Sea salt and freshly
 ground black pepper

For the rice

1 large sweet potato
2 tbsp garlic oil
175g/6oz white basmati
 rice
A small bunch of
 coriander
Sea salt and freshly
 ground black pepper

Vibrant in colour and intense in flavour, this dish will brighten up any autumnal day, however grey and chilly. The rice, with its 'croutons' of garlicky sweet potato, complements the aubergines beautifully. Highly versatile, it would make a lovely accompaniment to other dishes too – try it with stuffed peppers, tagines or roasted meats. I like to add chopped coriander to the rice, but any combination of fresh herbs would work.

Preheat the oven to 200°C/400°F/gas mark 6.

First prepare the sweet potato 'croutons' for the rice. Peel the sweet potato and trim the curved edges until you are left with a clean rectangular block, then cut into 5mm/¼in cubes. Place on a baking tray, drizzle with the garlic oil and season well with salt and pepper. Mix thoroughly and bake in the oven for 25–30 minutes or until the sweet potato cubes are golden and crunchy on the outside and soft in the middle. Remove from the oven and set aside.

Meanwhile, cut the aubergines in half lengthways and carefully scoop out the flesh. Using a food processor or sharp knife, finely chop the aubergine flesh so that it becomes almost pulpy. Finely dice the onion, cut the tomatoes into quarters and thinly slice the garlic cloves into rounds, then finely chop the mint and set aside.

Pour half the olive oil into a heavy-based pan and sauté the onion over a low heat for 5 minutes. Add the aubergine flesh, season with salt and pepper and continue to sauté gently for 10–15 minutes or until both the onions and aubergines are soft and slightly browned. Add the turmeric and ground coriander, mixing in thoroughly, and continue to cook over a low heat for a further 2 minutes. Remove from the heat and stir in the tomatoes and mint, seasoning further to taste.

Carefully rub the remaining olive oil into the aubergine skins and then fill with the aubergine mixture. Top each aubergine half with slices of garlic, spaced evenly apart, then cover loosely with foil and bake in the oven for 40 minutes.

Meanwhile, place the rice in a large saucepan with 500ml/18fl oz water and a pinch of salt, cover with a lid and bring to the boil. Once boiling, reduce the heat to low and simmer gently for about 10 minutes or until the rice has absorbed all the water. Using a fork, fluff up the cooked grains, then finely chop the coriander and add to the rice with the sweet potatoes, mixing in thoroughly and seasoning lightly with salt and pepper to taste. Remove the aubergines from the oven and serve with the rice.

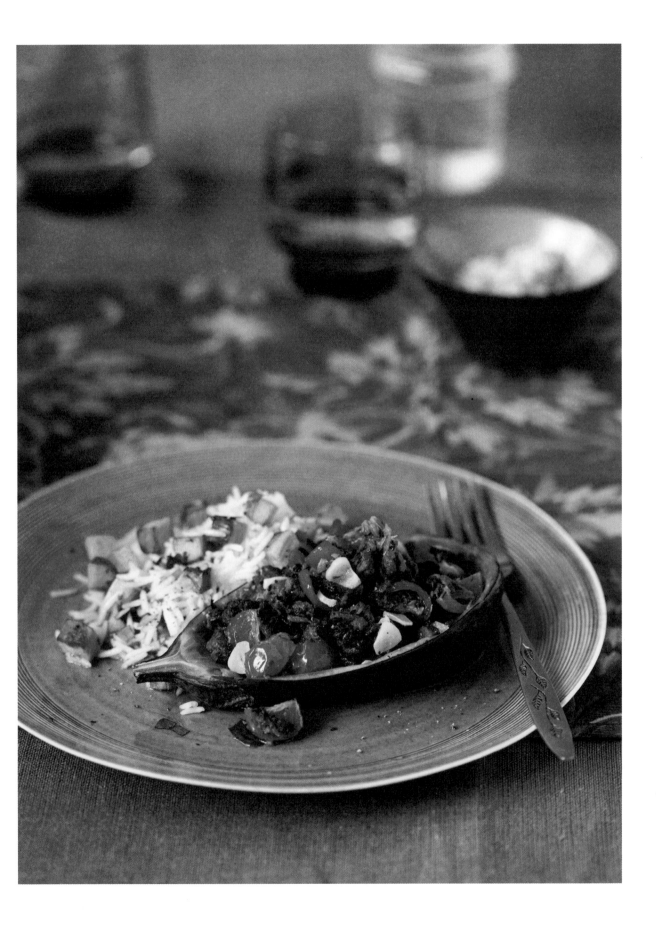

Wild Mushroom and Butternut Squash Risotto

Serves 4
Contains nuts

—

1 clove of garlic
250g/9oz wild mushrooms
2½ tbsp olive oil
1 small white onion
175g/6oz Arborio rice
2 rounded tsp Pure
   Sunflower Spread
   (dairy-free margarine)
A small bunch of curly-
   leaf parsley
Juice of ½ lemon
Sea salt and freshly
   ground black pepper

For the stock
1 butternut squash
1 tbsp olive oil
Sea salt and freshly
   ground black pepper

This risotto combines the earthy, nutty flavours of wild mushrooms with the natural sweetness of butternut squash. I personally favour a combination of porcini, chanterelles and perhaps a field mushroom or two. Roasting the squash before making it into stock adds a gorgeous depth of flavour but the art of making a good risotto lies in love and attention: take your time to stir in the stock and really tend to your dish.

Preheat the oven to 180°C/350°F/gas mark 4.

Begin by making the stock. Cut the butternut squash into quarters, leaving the skin on, and scoop out the seeds and fibres. Place on a baking tray, drizzle with the olive oil and season with salt and pepper, then roast in the oven for 45 minutes or until soft and tender to the point of a knife. Remove from the oven and allow to cool slightly.

Meanwhile, crush the garlic and tear the mushrooms into bite-sized pieces, then add both to a large bowl. Pour over 1 tablespoon of the olive oil, mix well and leave to marinate.

Once the squash has cooled slightly, remove the skin and cut the flesh into rough chunks. Add to a saucepan, cover with 1.2 litres/2 pints of water and bring to the boil, then reduce the heat to low and simmer for 10 minutes. Remove from the heat and, using a hand-held blender, blitz until you have a smooth light stock.

Next, finely dice the onion. Heat the remaining olive oil in a large, heavy-based saucepan and fry the onion over a low–medium heat for about 8 minutes or until soft but not browned. Add the rice and fry gently, stirring continuously, for approximately 2 minutes or until the rice has become glassy in appearance.

Begin to ladle in the stock, stirring constantly and ensuring that each ladleful has been absorbed before you add the next. Continue for 25–30 minutes or until nearly all the stock has been absorbed and the risotto is cooked through – the rice should be tender but still retain some bite. Add the margarine, season well with salt and pepper, cover with a lid and set aside (kept in the warm pan like this, the risotto will retain its heat) while you cook the mushrooms.

Heat a griddle pan or heavy-based frying pan until very hot, add the marinated mushrooms and cook for 2–3 minutes or until softened. Finely chop the parsley and add to a bowl with the fried mushrooms and the lemon juice, then season with salt and pepper and mix well. Spoon the risotto into large bowls and pile the herby garlic mushrooms on top to serve.

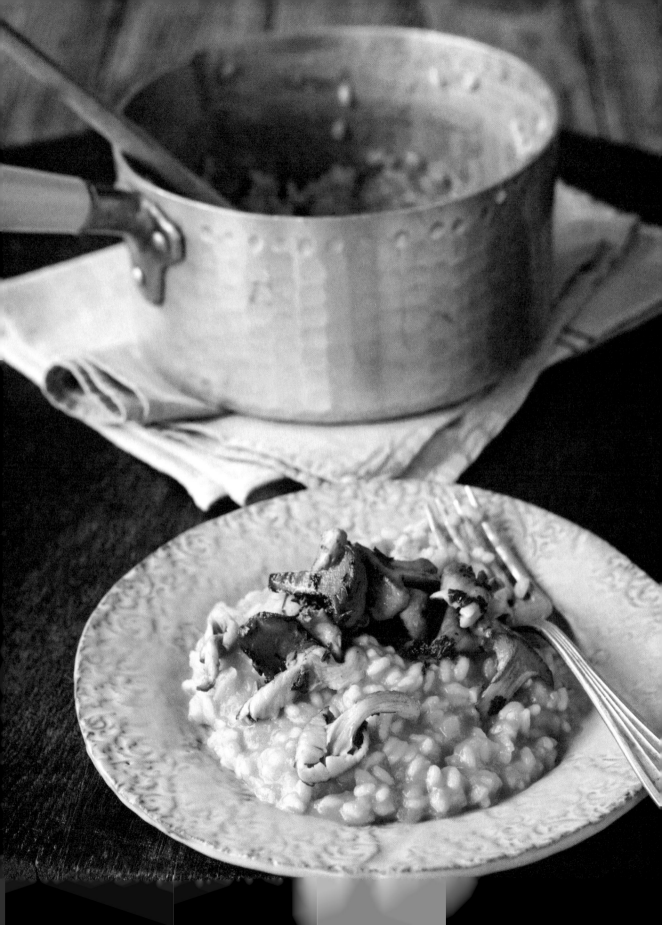

Plum and Oat Crunch with Honey Cream

Serves 4
Contains nuts

—

For the oat crunch
125g/4½oz porridge oats
½ tsp ground mixed spice
½ tsp ground cinnamon
75g/3oz demerara sugar
110g/4oz Pure Sunflower
 Spread (dairy-free
 margarine)

For the compote
1.25kg/2lb 12oz ripe
 plums
100ml/3½fl oz runny
 honey

For the honey cream
200g/7oz unsalted
 cashew nuts
2 tsp runny honey
150ml/5fl oz rice milk
¼ tsp vanilla extract

*You will need a shallow
18 x 28cm/7 x 11in baking
tin for this recipe*

A sweet little pudding in all senses of the word, the sweetness of the oat crunch and honey cream is complemented by the compote of tangy plums. It makes a wonderful light dessert but I also like to eat it for breakfast – it feels delightfully decadent. Present it layered in glass ramekins or even pretty teacups and saucers for a vintage tea-party feel. Try to layer the dish just before serving – or no longer than 2 hours ahead – as the granola can become slightly soggy from the plum juices. Once made, the plum compote and honey cream could be covered and kept in the fridge until ready to serve.

Preheat the oven to 190°C/375°F/gas mark 5 and lightly grease the baking tin.

Begin by making the honey cream. Place all the ingredients in a blender and pulse until completely smooth, thick and creamy – think the consistency of whipped double cream. If the mixture is a little grainy, continue to pulse until smooth, adding a little more rice milk if needed. Transfer to a bowl, cover and chill in the fridge for 1–2 hours.

Meanwhile, make the oat crunch. Combine the oats, spices and sugar in a large bowl, then melt the margarine in a small saucepan, pour over the oats and sugar and mix together.

Press the mixture over the base of the baking tin and bake in the oven for 15 minutes or until golden in colour. Remove from the oven and use a wooden spoon to break up the oat mixture into small clusters before allowing to cool down completely in the tin.

Meanwhile, make the compote. Halve the plums and remove the stones, then place in a large saucepan with the honey and 150ml/5fl oz water and bring to the boil. Once boiling, reduce the heat to low and simmer for 3–4 minutes or until the plums are just tender to the point of a knife. Drain almost all of the syrup from the plums, reserving a third of it, and set aside to cool down.

Once cool, divide half of the plums between four ramekins or other dishes of your choice, layering the stewed fruit across the bottom and pouring over a little of the reserved syrup (just enough to coat the plums). Cover with a layer of the oat crunch and then add the remaining plums to make another layer. Top with a final layer of the oat crunch and a drizzle of the syrup. Cover and chill in the fridge for no longer than 2 hours (or make up the dish just before serving – see the introduction) until ready to serve and then top with a large spoonful of honey cream and a final sprinkling of the oat crunch.

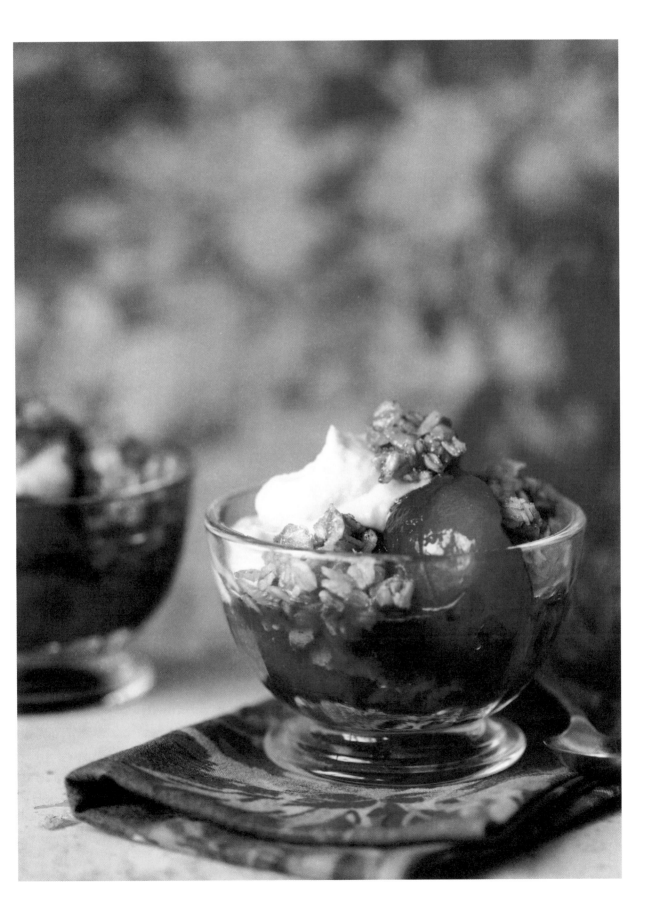

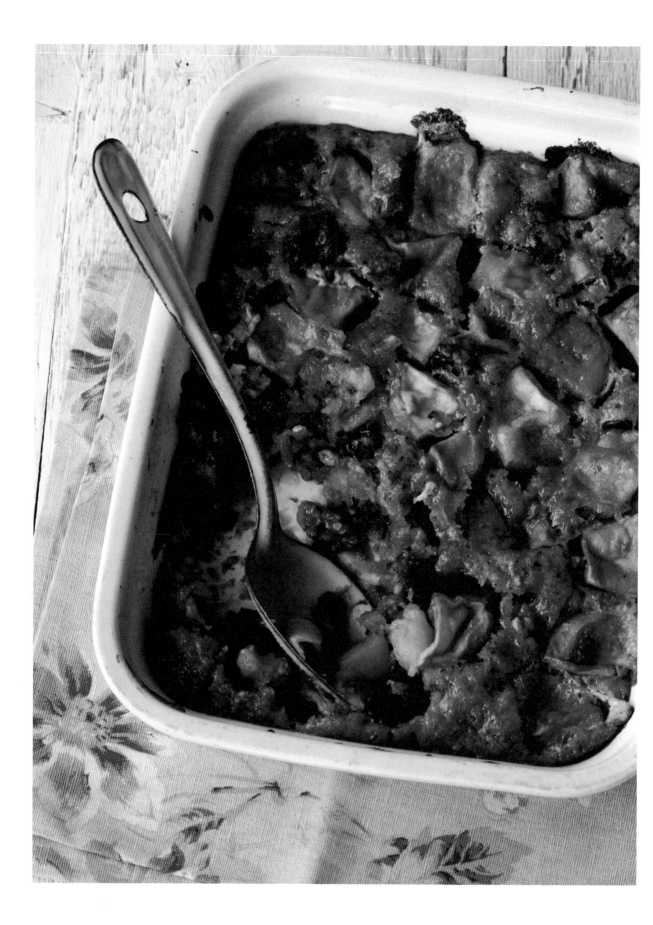

Baked Apple Charlotte

Serves 6
Contains nuts

—

2 tbsp Pure Sunflower
  Spread (dairy-free
  margarine), plus extra
  for greasing
75g/3oz pitted medjool
  dates
60g/2oz shelled walnuts
450g/1lb Bramley cooking
  apples
110g/4oz gluten-free
  self-raising flour
  (ideally Doves Farm)
125ml/4fl oz rice milk
1 heaped tsp egg replacer
  (ideally Orgran) whisked
  with 2 tbsp water
175g/6oz soft light brown
  sugar

*You will need a shallow
ovenproof dish,
approximately 10 x
20cm/4 x 8in in size,
for this recipe*

*I love this combination of ingredients – apples mixed with brown sugar,
dried fruit and nuts – in all its guises, whether crumbles, strudels or
simple baked apples. Of them all, however, this pudding has to be my
absolute favourite, with the dates adding an irresistibly gooey, brownie-
like texture. It's easy to make and wonderful served hot with a pouring of
oat cream or custard (see page 208). It's also delicious eaten cold, cut into
slices and enjoyed as a treat – bear that in mind if there's any left!*

Preheat the oven to 200°C/400°F/gas mark 6 and lightly grease the
ovenproof dish.

Chop the dates and walnuts into small pieces, then peel and core
the apples and cut into 2cm/¾in chunks.

Melt the margarine in a small saucepan and sift the flour into a
large bowl, making a well in the centre. Pour the melted margarine
into the flour with the rice milk and the egg replacer mixture and beat
together until you have a smooth and glossy batter (add a dash more
milk if you think it necessary), and then continue to beat lightly for
another 1–2 minutes.

Add the sugar, dates, walnuts and apples to the batter and mix
thoroughly before pouring into the ovenproof dish. Spread the mixture
evenly in the dish and bake in the oven for 45–50 minutes until golden
and cooked through (a skewer or cocktail stick inserted into the centre
of the pudding should come out clean). Remove from the oven and
serve while hot.

Pecan Pie

Serves 8
Contains nuts

—

1 quantity of sweet
  Shortcrust Pastry
  (see page 223) with
  the addition of 1 tsp of
  cinammon in step 1

For the filling
190g/6½oz soft
  dark brown sugar
125ml/4½fl oz maple
  syrup
30g/1¼oz Pure
  Sunflower Spread
  (dairy-free margarine)
200g/7oz shelled pecan
  nuts
6 tbsp ground flaxseeds
½ tsp baking powder
1 tsp vanilla extract
A pinch of salt

*You will need a 23cm/9in
deep-fluted tart tin with
a removable base for this
recipe*

*With its rich shortcrust base and voluptuous, sweet filling, pecan pie
must be the ultimate in decadence. And there can surely be nothing more
enticing in both taste and aroma than this pie, freshly baked and straight
from the oven. The combination of maple syrup and dark brown sugar
gives real intensity to the flavour, while the ground flaxseeds (replacing
eggs in the recipe) add extra texture to the filling. This is a pie for sharing,
so invite everyone round and tuck in!*

First make the filling. Place the sugar in a saucepan with the maple syrup
and margarine and bring to the boil. Boil the mixture for 1 minute,
stirring constantly, then remove from the heat and set aside to cool
down for about 15 minutes – but not much longer or the syrup will set.

Meanwhile, roughly chop the pecan nuts and, in a separate bowl,
mix together the ground flaxseeds and baking powder with 9 tablespoons
of water to form a thick paste. (The mixture will get thicker and thicker
the longer you leave it, but don't worry as this is meant to happen.)

Preheat the oven to 180°C/350°F/gas mark 4 and place a baking
sheet into the oven to preheat.

Roll out the cinnamon pastry and fill the tart tin following the
instructions given in the Shortcrust Pastry recipe on page 223.

Next stir the flaxseed mixture into the cooled syrup with the vanilla
extract and salt, mixing together until smooth, then stir in the chopped
pecans. Pour the filling into the tart case, levelling the surface with the
back of your spoon, and bake in the oven on the preheated baking sheet
for 35–40 minutes or until the filling has just set and is still a tiny bit
wobbly in the middle. Leave the pie in its tin on a wire rack to cool for
10 minutes before serving with a spoonful of oat cream or Vanilla Ice
Cream (see page 66).

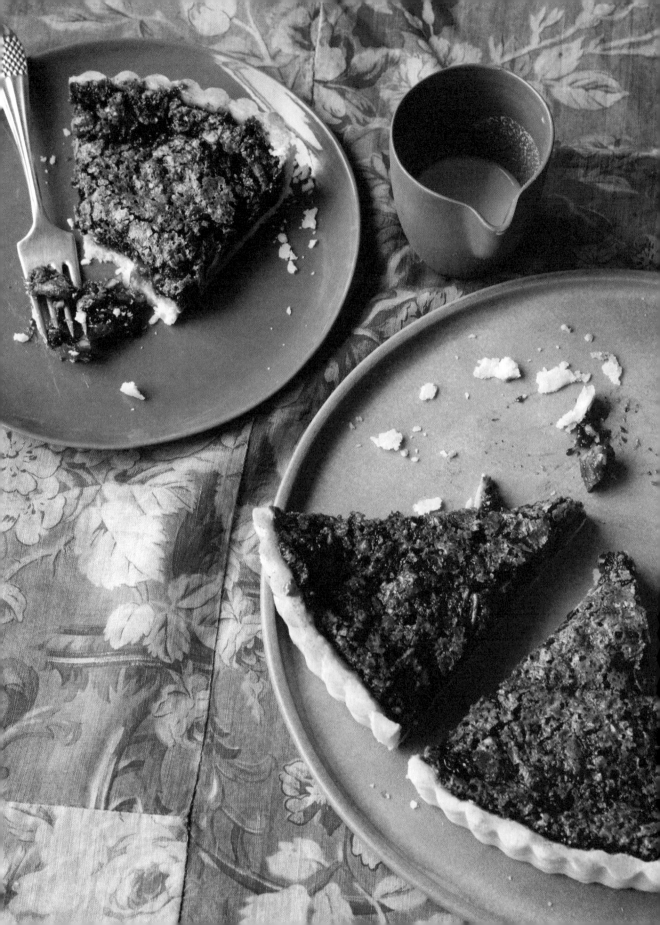

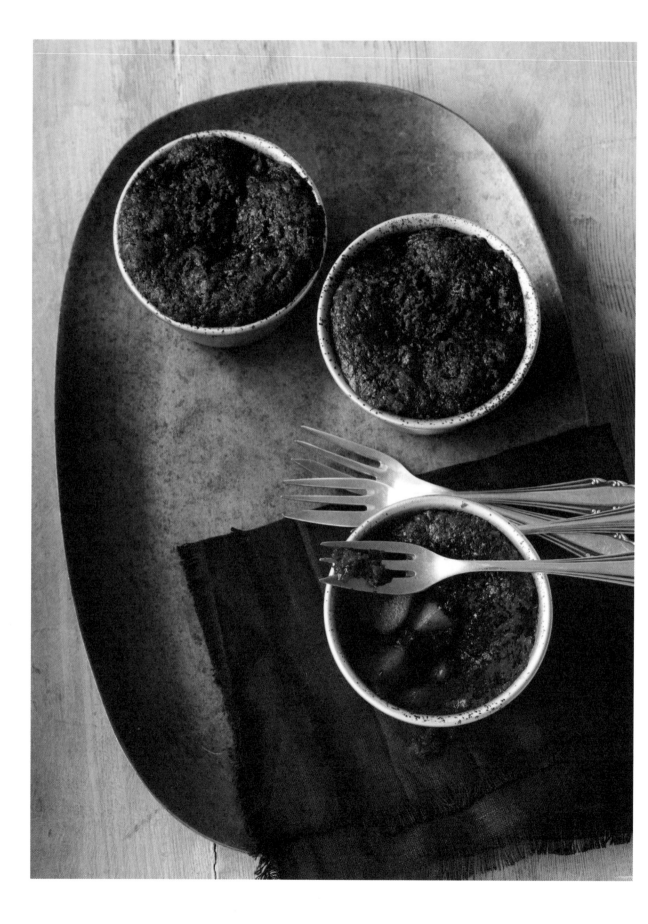

Chocolate and Pear Puddings

Makes 4 puddings

—

50g/1¾oz Pure
  Sunflower Spread
  (dairy-free margarine),
  plus extra for greasing
2 tbsp ground flaxseeds
⅛ tsp baking powder
2 ripe pears
100g/3½oz gluten-free
  self-raising flour
  (ideally Doves Farm)
2 tbsp cocoa powder,
  plus extra for dusting
125g/4oz golden caster
  sugar
6 tbsp rice milk
4 heaped tsp soft dark
  brown sugar
4 tbsp boiling water

*You will need four 8cm/
3in diameter ramekins
for this recipe*

Pear and chocolate work wonderfully well together and these individual puddings are a real treat to eat. The top of the pudding produces a light crunch as you bite into it, giving way to a rich chocolaty centre, studded with little bursts of tender, juicy pear. Always use pears that are good for eating raw, such as Comice, as well as fairly ripe, as this makes all the difference to the flavour.

Preheat the oven to 180°C/350°F/gas mark 4 and lightly grease the ramekins.

Place the ground flaxseeds and baking powder in a small bowl and mix with 3 tablespoons of water, then set aside to thicken while you peel and core the pears and chop them into 1.5cm/⅝in chunks.

Next melt the margarine in a small saucepan over a low heat, then remove from the heat and allow to cool but not set.

Sift the flour and the cocoa powder into a large bowl, then tip in the caster sugar and stir together. Place the melted margarine and the flaxseed mixture in a separate bowl, add the rice milk and whisk until combined. Pour into the flour and sugar and continue to whisk together until smooth, then fold in the pear pieces.

Spoon the mixture into the ramekins and place on a baking tray. Evenly sprinkle the brown sugar and a little extra cocoa powder over each pudding, followed by 1 tablespoon of boiling water. Place in the oven and cook for 25 minutes or until a cocktail stick inserted in the centre of each pudding comes out clean. Serve while they are still warm.

Apple and Blackberry Cake

Serves 8

—

110g/4oz Pure Sunflower Spread (dairy-free margarine), plus extra for greasing

225g/8oz gluten-free self-raising flour (ideally Doves Farm)

½ tsp baking powder

1 tsp mixed spice

1 tsp ground cinnamon

110g/4oz soft light brown sugar

2 rounded tbsp apple purée (for homemade, see page 16)

2 large Bramley cooking apples

100g/3½oz fresh or frozen blackberries

3 tbsp rice milk

You will need a 20cm/ 8in diameter cake tin with a removable base for this recipe

Autumn really lends itself to baking – the sublime smells wafting through your home can make everything seem right with the world. Now is the time to find British apples in abundance, making this cake the ideal afternoon treat. Sweet and moist and spiced with cinnamon, the sponge is dotted with tangy nuggets of apple and blackberry. The texture is divinely moist and light due to the inclusion of apple purée as a replacement for the eggs, and it goes down equally well for afternoon tea or dessert, served slightly warmed with a scoop of Vanilla Ice Cream or a spoonful of Honey Cream (see pages 66 and 154).

Preheat the oven to 190°C/375°F/gas mark 5, then lightly grease the cake tin and line the base with baking parchment.

Sift the flour into a large bowl with the baking powder, mixed spice and ground cinnamon and mix in the sugar. Dice the margarine and rub in with the apple purée until the mixture forms soft clumps.

Peel and core the apples and dice into 1cm/½in cubes. Fold the chopped apple and the blackberries into the cake mixture, ensuring that they are evenly distributed.

Now pour in the rice milk, one tablespoon at a time and mixing carefully as you go, until the cake mixture pulls together and forms a batter. (You may need to add a little extra or a little less rice milk, so play it by eye.)

Tip the cake mixture into the prepared tin and bake for 30–40 minutes or until risen, firm to the touch and golden in colour. Transfer to a wire rack and leave the cake to cool in its tin for 10 minutes before turning out and serving.

Sticky Date Squares

Makes 12 slices
—
175g/6oz Pure
  Sunflower Spread
  (dairy-free margarine),
  plus extra for greasing
200g/7oz pitted dates
175g/6oz gluten-free plain
  flour (ideally Doves Farm)
1/2 tsp bicarbonate
  of soda
A pinch of salt
175g/6oz soft light brown
  sugar
100g/3½oz jumbo
  porridge oats

*You will need a 20cm/8in
square baking tin for this
recipe*

*This recipe instantly transports me back to my childhood and memories of
my first taste of dates (figs also come to mind) – fascinatingly sweet on the
tongue and wonderfully gooey in texture. Here the dates are cooked into a
delectable sticky paste and then sandwiched between two layers of golden
crumbly oats. Stored in an airtight container, they will last for up to a week
– if you can resist them for that long. Alternatively, they freeze very well.*

Preheat the oven to 180°C/350°F/gas mark 4, then lightly grease
the baking tin and line the base with baking parchment.

Roughly chop the dates and place in a saucepan with 250ml/9fl oz
water. Bring to a gentle simmer and cook for 15 minutes, uncovered and
over a low–medium heat, stirring occasionally, until the dates have
formed a soft and thick paste. Remove from the heat and set aside to cool.

Meanwhile, sift the flour, bicarbonate of soda and salt into a large
bowl and then stir in the sugar and oats. Dice the margarine into small
cubes and add to the bowl, rubbing it in with your fingertips until you
have a crumble-like mixture forming soft clumps.

Press half of the oat mixture into the base of the prepared tin so that
if forms an even layer. Spread the cooled date paste over this and then
sprinkle with the remaining oat mixture, pressing very lightly with the
palm of your hand to flatten the top of the mixture.

Bake in the oven for 40 minutes or until golden brown and set in
the middle. (You can test this by inserting a cocktail stick or skewer into
the centre of the date mixture: if it comes out clean then the mixture is
cooked, but if there are clumps of uncooked mixture attached to it, then
pop the tin back in the oven for a few more minutes before testing
again.) Remove from the oven and transfer the tin to a wire rack,
allowing the date mixture to cool down completely before cutting into
squares and removing from the tin.

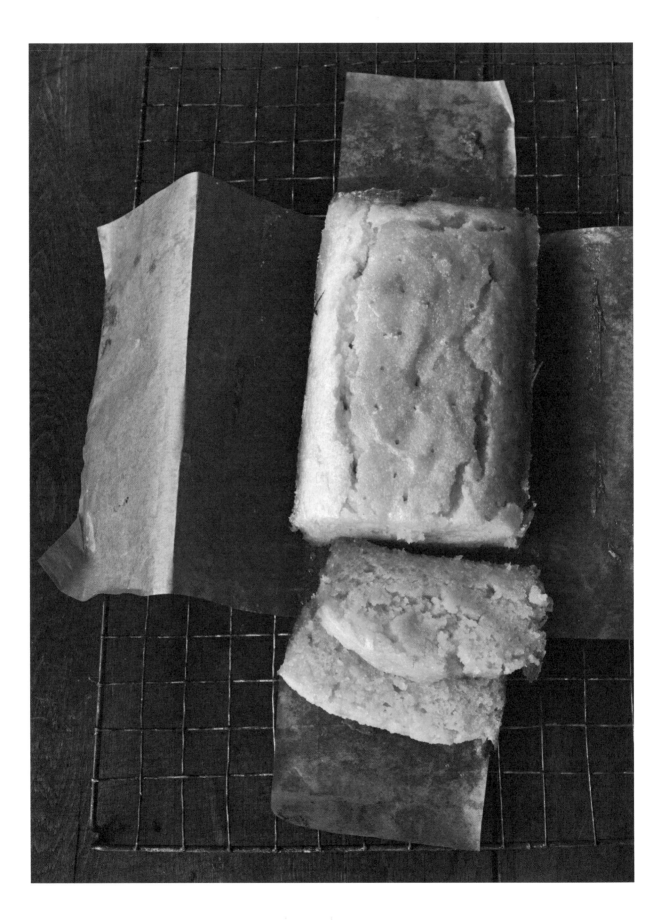

Lemon Drizzle Cake

Serves 8

—

225g/8oz Pure Sunflower Spread (dairy-free margarine), plus extra for greasing

225g/8oz golden caster sugar

4 heaped tsp egg replacer (ideally Orgran) whisked with 8 tbsp water

225g/8oz gluten-free self-raising flour (ideally Doves Farm)

1 tsp xanthan gum

Grated zest of 1 lemon

1 tbsp rice milk

For the lemon drizzle

75g/3oz golden caster sugar

Juice of 1½ lemons

You will need a 900g/2lb loaf tin for this recipe

Good lemon drizzle cake tastes heaven sent and this particular version is worth its weight in sugary, lemony gold. I love to serve it on a warm afternoon with a pot of tea and lots of friends to ooh and ah over it. It will stay fresh for a few days in a sealed tin and also freezes very well, keeping for up to a month.

Preheat the oven to 180°C/350°F/gas mark 4, then grease the loaf tin and line the base and sides with baking parchment.

Cream the margarine and sugar together gently with a wooden spoon until pale and fluffy, then add the egg replacer mixture, a bit at a time, slowly stirring it in until fully combined.

Sift in the flour and xanthan gum, then add the lemon zest and rice milk. Mix well until fully incorporated and then spoon into the lined loaf tin, levelling the top of the cake with the back of your spoon.

Bake in the oven for 45–50 minutes or until cooked through and a skewer or cocktail stick inserted into the centre of the cake comes out clean. Allow the cake to cool a little in its tin while you mix together the sugar and lemon juice to drizzle over the cake.

Pierce the warm cake all over using the skewer or a fork and then pour over the sweetened lemon juice. This will be absorbed into the cake, forming a sugary crust on the cake's surface as it dries. Leave the cake in its tin until completely cool and then cut into slices to serve.

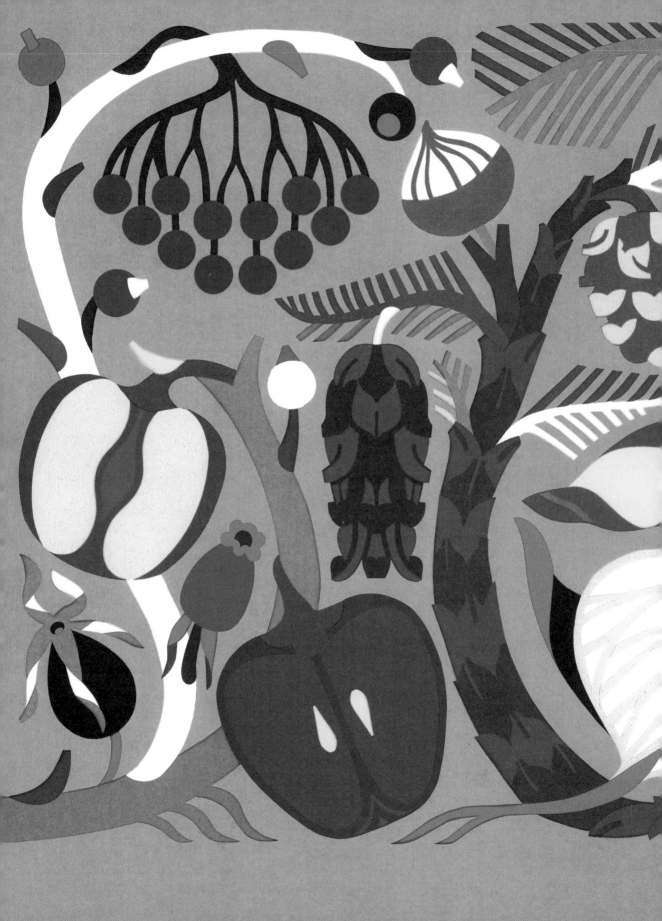

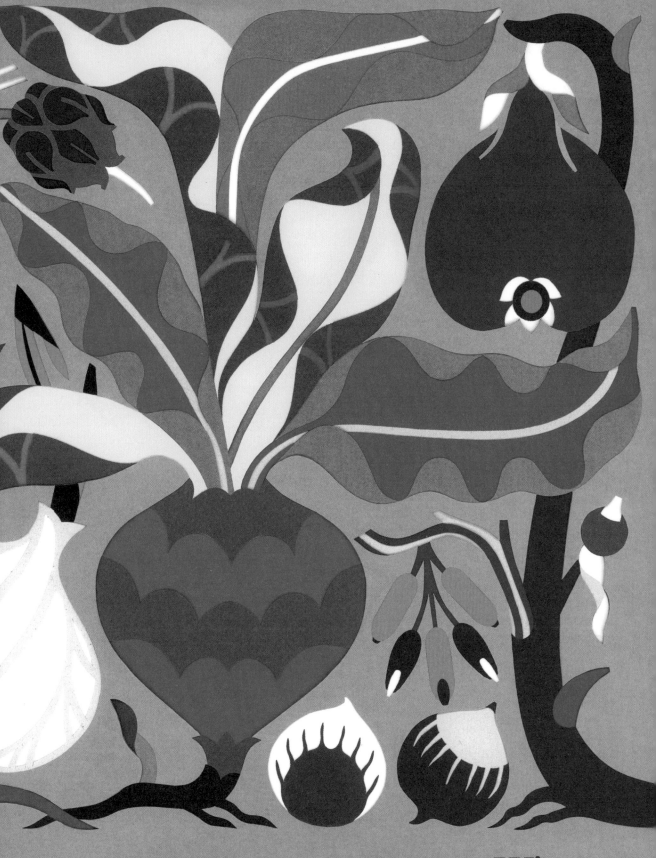

Winter

Moody skies and biting air call for the comfort of warming and hearty foods. This is the season of sustaining meals – steaming soups and stews, hot pies and rich puddings. Dishes such as Baked Apple and Mustard Ham with Parsnip Purée or Roast Beef with Horseradish Cream and Olive Oil Mashed Potato (see pages 182, 184 and 192) use the best of the starch-sweet winter roots for a fortifying lunch. For those who don't eat meat, Vegetable Lasagne (see page 199) is creamy and comforting, a perfect suppertime dish, while Little Sticky Toffee Puddings (see page 206) will satisfy those sweet cravings, wrapping you in warmth for the chilly weeks ahead.

Roasted Pepper and Lentil Soup

Serves 4

—

2 red peppers

2 large tomatoes

2 tbsp olive oil

1 tsp soft light brown
  sugar

2 x 400g tins of chopped
  tomatoes

1 tsp harissa paste
  (for homemade, see
  page 148)

1 x 400g tin of lentils,
  drained and rinsed

A small bunch of flat-leaf
  parsley

Sea salt and freshly
  ground black pepper

This soup has many virtues: the rich colour, the sweet smokiness of the roasted peppers and the sustaining comfort of the lentils. Plus, and this is not a minor detail, it is really simple to make, using chiefly storecupboard ingredients. We all have days when the idea of peeling, blanching, wrapping, trussing and baking all seem like too much effort. Those are the times when dishes like this soup really come into their own. A meal in itself, it just needs a hunk of my Crusty White Loaf (see page 218) to accompany it for a satisfying meal.

Preheat the oven to 200°C/400°F/gas mark 6.

Deseed the peppers and chop into 5cm/2in chunks, then quarter the fresh tomatoes. Place the peppers and tomatoes in a roasting tin, combine with the olive oil and sugar and season well with salt and pepper. Place in the oven and bake for 30 minutes or until the peppers and tomatoes are soft and slightly charred.

Meanwhile, in a large saucepan mix together the tinned tomatoes and harissa paste. Once the peppers are cooked, add them to the saucepan with a third of the lentils and, using a food processor or hand-held blender, blitz until smooth. Add the remaining lentils to the soup, season well with salt and pepper and heat through at a gentle simmer for 10 minutes. Chop the parsley and sprinkle over the finished soup to serve.

Roast Butternut Squash, Coconut and Chilli Soup

Serves 4
Contains nuts

—

1kg/2lb 3oz butternut
   squash
4 cloves of garlic
1 large onion
A small bunch of
   coriander
1 tsp chilli flakes
2 tsp ground cumin
2 tsp ground coriander
3 tbsp groundnut or
   rapeseed oil
2 tsp soft light brown
   sugar
1.2 litres/2 pints
   vegetable stock
200ml/7fl oz coconut
   milk
Sea salt and freshly
   ground black pepper

A cold winter's day demands a steaming bowl of soup and this luxuriant, fiery dish is a real winter warmer: the sweetness of the roasted butternut squash is given a sizzling boost by the chilli, which then melds into the cooling and velvety-smooth coconut milk. It makes for a truly delicious lunch or supper and will warm the coldest of bones.

Preheat the oven to 200°C/400°F/gas mark 6.

Slice the butternut squash in half lengthways, scooping out the seeds and fibres and discarding these. Peel the squash halves and chop into small chunks. Crush the garlic and roughly chop the onion, then finely chop the fresh coriander and set aside.

Place the butternut squash in a roasting tin with the chilli flakes, ground spices and 2 tablespoons of the groundnut or rapeseed oil and mix together so that the chunks of squash are well coated in the spicy oil. Season with salt and pepper and roast in the oven for 45–50 minutes, stirring occasionally, until the butternut squash is soft and tender and slightly caramelised.

Meanwhile, pour the remaining groundnut or rapeseed oil into a large saucepan, add the onion, garlic and sugar and sauté over the lowest heat for about 25 minutes or until soft and golden.

Add the roasted squash to the onions – scraping out all of the spice from the roasting tin to add to the pan – and pour over the vegetable stock. Heat the soup until simmering, then remove from the heat and stir in the coconut milk. Using a food processor or hand-held blender, blitz until smooth and velvety in consistency. Heat the soup through, season with salt and pepper to taste and ladle into bowls. Serve hot with a sprinkling of chopped coriander on each bowl.

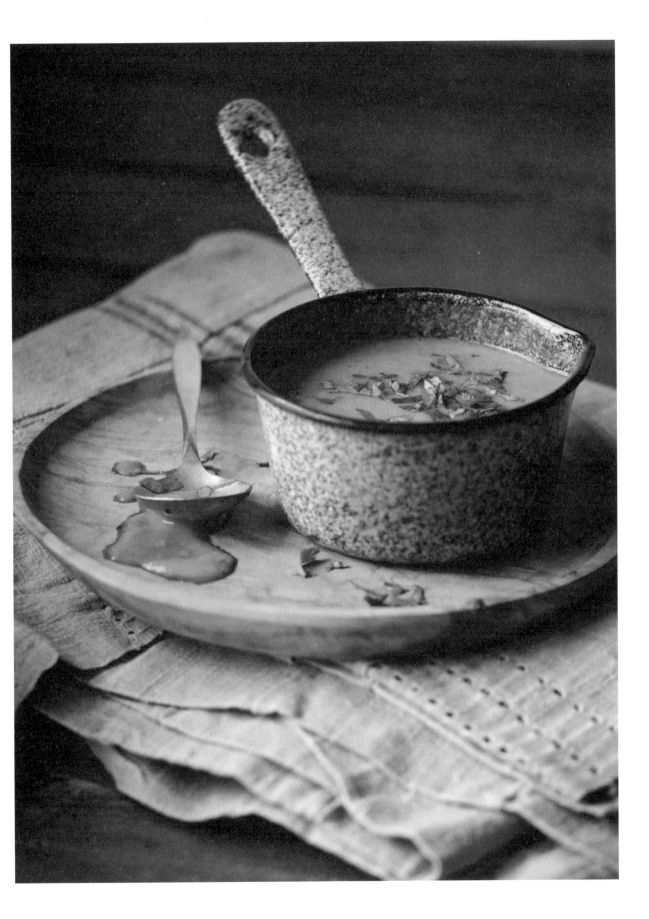

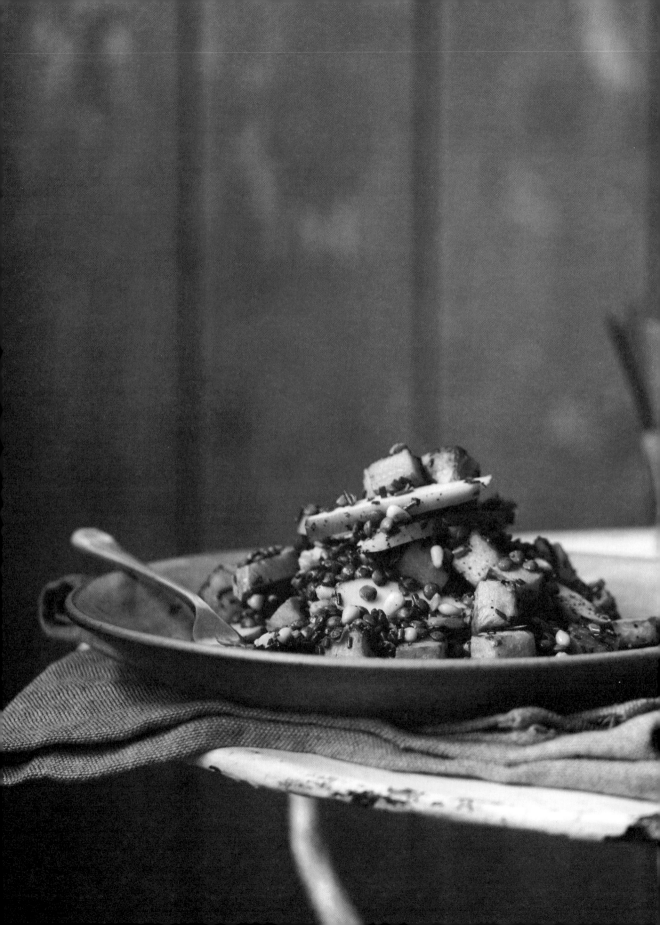

Smoked Chicken, Sweet Potato and Lentil Salad

Serves 4
Contains nuts

—

700g/1½lb sweet
    potatoes
2 smoked chicken breasts
3 cloves of garlic
A bunch of chives
3 tbsp olive oil
50g/1¾oz pine nuts
250g/9oz Puy lentils
Sea salt and freshly
    ground black pepper

For the dressing
2 tbsp extra-virgin
    olive oil
1 tbsp lemon juice
2 tsp agave syrup or 1 tsp
    soft light brown sugar
Sea salt and freshly
    ground black pepper

This is a glorious salad for a winter's day: the earthy Puy lentils and cubes of roasted garlicky sweet potato mingling with the mellow and smoky flavour of the chicken and the crunch of pine nuts. You can buy ready-smoked chicken in good delis and quality butchers, as well as some supermarkets, and it is well worth hunting down; but if you can't find any, then seasoned, cooked chicken breasts will work well too.

Preheat the oven to 220°C/425°F/gas mark 7.

Peel the sweet potatoes and trim the curved edges of each potato until you are left with a clean rectangular block. (You can freeze the trimmed parts and use them in stocks or soups at a later date.) Chop the sweet potato blocks into cubes exactly 1cm/½in square.

Slice the smoked chicken into small chunks approximately 1.5cm/⅝in in size, then crush the garlic and finely chop the chives. Place the sweet potato in a roasting tin and combine with the olive oil and crushed garlic, season well with salt and pepper and roast in the oven for 35 minutes or until softened on the inside, crisp on the outside and golden brown at the edges. Once cooked, remove from the oven and set aside.

Meanwhile, scatter the pine nuts on a baking sheet and toast in the oven, turning them occasionally to make sure they don't burn, for 5–6 minutes or until golden brown. Remove from the oven and set aside to cool down.

While the sweet potatoes are still cooking, place the lentils in a large saucepan and pour over enough water to cover them by at least 8cm/3in. Bring to the boil, then reduce the heat to low and simmer uncovered for 20–25 minutes or until the lentils are just tender, adding more water if necessary.

Next make the dressing by mixing all the ingredients together in a bowl, seasoning with salt and pepper and whisking with a fork to amalgamate the flavours.

Once the lentils are cooked, drain and place in a serving bowl, pour over the dressing and stir well, seasoning further to taste and adding more olive oil if you think it needs it. Tip in the roasted sweet potato, smoked chicken, pine nuts and chopped chives, toss carefully to mix together and serve while warm, ideally on a bed of watercress or lettuce leaves.

Hot-smoked Salmon Pâté

Serves 4

—

½ small red onion

A small bunch of
curly-leaf parsley

300g/11oz hot-smoked
salmon

2 tsp English mustard
(2 heaped tsp mustard
powder mixed with
2 tsp water)

2 tbsp oat cream

1 tsp agave syrup

1 tbsp lemon juice

Sea salt and freshly
ground black pepper

'Hot-smoking' is the Scandinavian way of smoking fish – the salmon is smoked at a much hotter temperature for a shorter period of time, creating a flakier, lighter fillet that's slightly barbecued in flavour. Here, the salmon is blitzed with mustard, oat cream and parsley to make a wonderfully rich pâté. You could serve it as a starter or for a relaxed light lunch, with some of my Rye Soda Bread (see page 214), fresh from the oven. Equally, you could transform it into something a little more sophisticated by spreading it onto circles of rye toast and serving as a canapé with drinks. You can even prepare it the day ahead for a truly stress-free beginning to your evening. Once made, the pâté will keep for up to three days in the fridge.

Finely chop the onion and parsley and peel the skin from the smoked salmon. Place half the salmon in a food processor or blender with the chopped onion, mustard, oat cream, agave syrup and lemon juice and blend until smooth.

Break up the remaining salmon into small flakes and stir into the blended pâté with a grinding of pepper and the chopped parsley. Season with salt and more pepper to taste, adding more lemon juice if you think it needs it. Cover and chill in the fridge for at least an hour before serving.

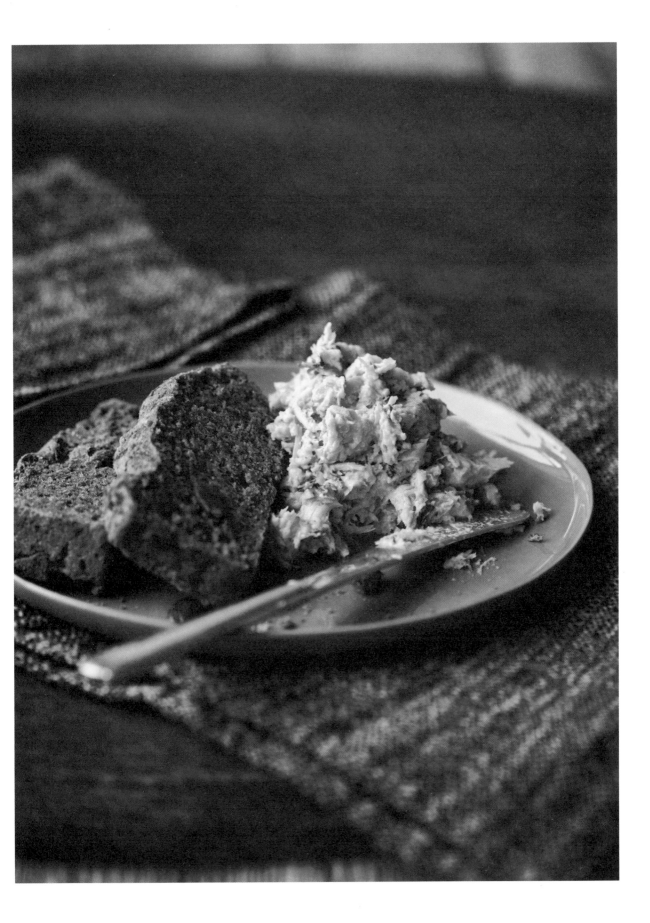

Salmon and Horseradish Fishcakes

Makes 4 fishcakes

—

400g/14oz floury potatoes
(such as Maris Piper)
75g/3oz fresh horseradish
1 tbsp dairy-free
margarine (ideally Pure
Sunflower Spread)
A small bunch of flat-leaf
parsley
200g/7oz cooked salmon
fillet
2 tbsp small capers,
drained and rinsed
1 tbsp groundnut
or rapeseed oil
Sea salt and freshly
ground black pepper

Fresh horseradish has a wonderful (and powerful) flavour hidden beneath its gnarled skin, a taste that I, personally, am addicted to. When you buy it fresh (from the market or a greengrocer) it usually comes as a large, whole root. My top tip would be to peel it and cut into 5cm/2in lengths, which you can then freeze. This means that whenever you need some horseradish – for making into a sauce (see page 192), for instance, or adding to mashed potato or these lovely fishcakes – you can simply take it from the freezer and grate it straight into your dish. Salmon and horseradish make a lovely pairing – serve on a bed of fresh watercress with a little grated beetroot, a wedge of lemon and a scattering of freshly milled black pepper. These fishcakes are ideal as a starter for four people, or they would make a delicious lunch for two.

Peel and cut the potatoes into 5cm/2in chunks. Place in a saucepan of salted water (the water should cover the potatoes by a couple of centimetres), then bring to the boil, reduce the heat and simmer uncovered for 10–15 minutes or until completely soft to the point of a knife. Once cooked, drain, season well with salt and pepper and mash until smooth, then set aside to cool slightly.

Peel and finely grate the horseradish and add to the potatoes with the margarine, mixing together until the horseradish is evenly distributed. Finely chop the parsley and break up the salmon into flakes, then stir into the potatoes with the capers. Season well with salt and pepper and mix everything together thoroughly so that the ingredients bind together.

Next carefully shape the potato mixture into four cakes, each approximately 8cm/3in in diameter (it helps if your hands are very cold or lightly floured), then cover and chill in the fridge for a minimum of 30 minutes.

When ready to cook, heat the groundnut or rapeseed oil in a non-stick frying pan and add the fishcakes. Fry gently for about 5 minutes on each side or until golden brown all over, then remove from the pan and serve immediately.

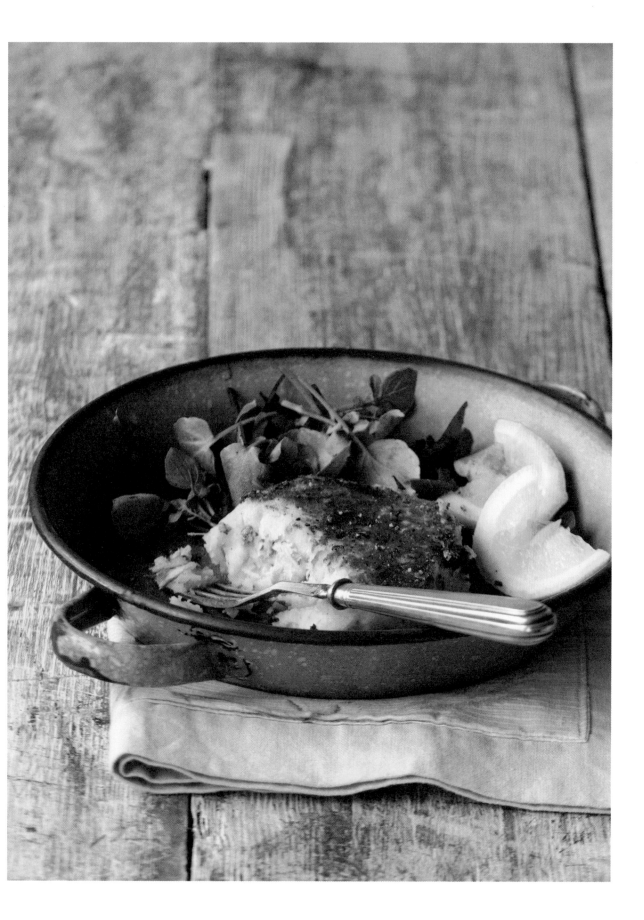

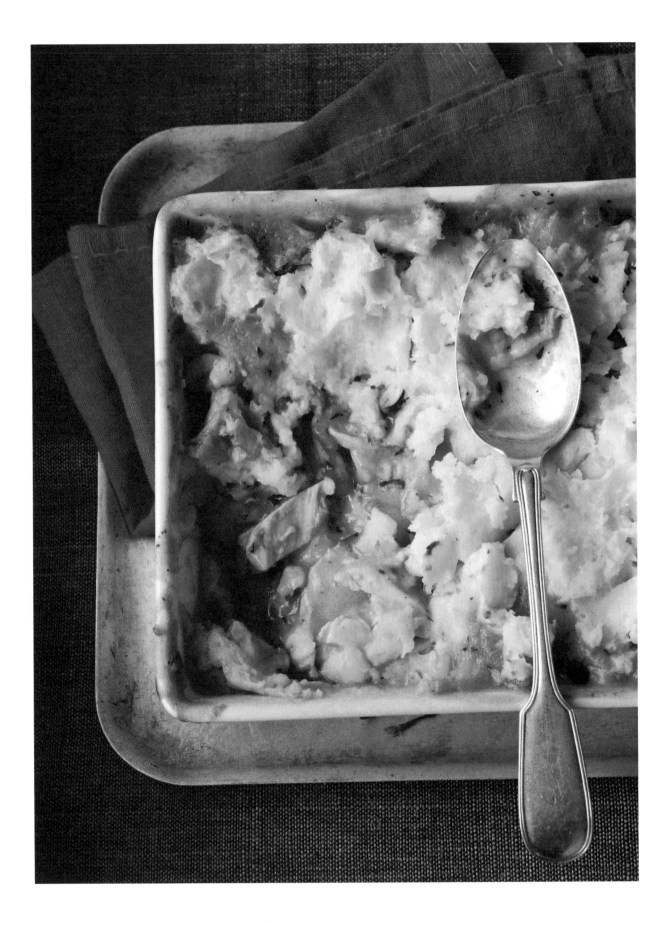

Chicken and Mushroom Pie

Serves 4

—

1 x 2kg/4lb 4½oz whole cooked chicken

1 large white onion

175g/6oz chestnut mushrooms

Leaves from 4 sprigs of thyme

Leaves from a small bunch of marjoram

125g/4½oz Pure Sunflower Spread (dairy-free margarine)

75g/3oz gluten-free plain flour (ideally Doves Farm)

1 bay leaf

500ml/18fl oz chicken stock

1.25kg/2lb 12oz floury potatoes

Sea salt and freshly ground black pepper

You will need a 23 x 30cm/ 9 x 12in ovenproof dish or 25cm/10in diameter pie dish for this recipe

This is effectively a traditional chicken and mushroom pie but with a topping of mashed potato rather than pastry. It must be the ultimate comfort food: perfect for a cold winter's day, robust enough to satisfy the largest of appetites while still being delicately flavoured. It's also as soothing to prepare as it is to eat. Serve it with a medley of vegetables – steamed broccoli and kale, caramelised carrots, garden peas and spiced red cabbage – plus a spoonful of redcurrant jelly for a glorious winter feast.

Preheat the oven to 200°C/400°F/gas mark 6.

Begin by cutting up the chicken – I recommend starting with the breasts and working down towards the legs. Remove any skin or excess fat from the meat and discard the remaining carcass or freeze to make stock from it at a later date. Chop the chicken meat into roughly 2.5cm/1in chunks and set aside.

Halve the onion and slice into thin half-moons, then cut the mushrooms into slices 5mm/¼in thick. Melt 75g/3oz of the margarine in a large saucepan, then add the onion, mushrooms and fresh herbs and season well with salt and pepper. Cover with a lid and cook over a very low heat for around 10 minutes or until soft and the onion is beginning to become translucent but not browned.

Add the flour to the onion and mushrooms and stir continuously over a low heat for 1 minute, so that the margarine and flour amalgamate and form a roux. Add the bay leaf and a little stock to the sauce and stir until the liquid is completely absorbed.

Repeat with the remaining stock, adding it bit by bit and stirring continuously, until it has all been amalgamated and the sauce is smooth. Once the sauce has thickened, bring to a simmer and stir constantly for 1 minute before taking off the heat. Remove the bay leaf and add the cooked chicken to the sauce, season with salt and pepper to taste and set aside.

Peel and cut the potatoes into 2.5cm/1in cubes. Place in a large saucepan of salted water (the water should cover the potatoes by a couple of centimetres) and bring to the boil, then reduce the heat and simmer uncovered for 10–15 minutes or until completely soft to the point of a knife. Drain and season liberally with salt and pepper, add the remaining margarine and mash until smooth and creamy.

Spoon the chicken and mushroom filling into your ovenproof dish and top evenly with the mashed potato. Place on a large baking sheet and cook in the oven for 30 minutes or until golden brown and bubbling on top.

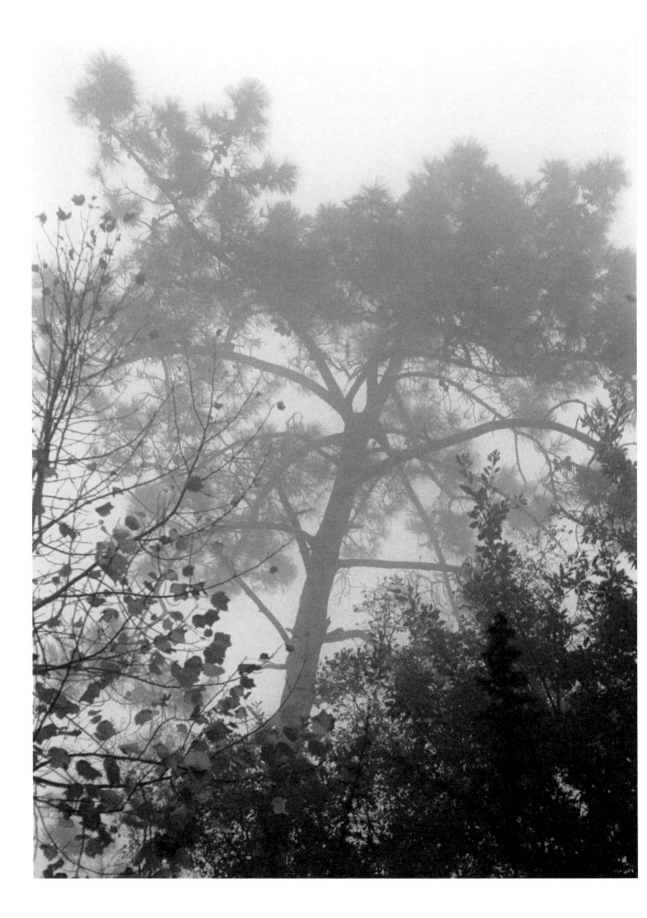

Clay Pot Chicken with Date and Nut Quinoa Stuffing

Serves 6
Contains nuts
—
1 x 2.5kg/5½lb chicken
1 tsp cumin seeds
1 tsp fennel seeds
25g/1oz pine nuts
1 red onion
2 cloves of garlic
1 tbsp olive oil
175g/6oz quinoa
500ml/18fl oz chicken
   stock
A small bunch of
   flat-leaf parsley
4 pitted dates
Juice of 1 lemon
40g/1½oz dairy-free
   margarine (ideally Pure
   Sunflower Spread)
Sea salt and freshly
   ground black pepper

You will need a terracotta chicken brick, pre-soaked for 20 minutes in cold water, or a large casserole dish for this recipe

This is the ultimate roast chicken. It is filled with an amazing stuffing – glossy light quinoa, soft dates and crunchy pine nuts blended with spices in a warming mix that's just right for the time of year. Based on the ancient technique of cooking in an earthenware container over an open fire, a chicken brick is essentially a clay oven within an oven. If you don't have one just use a large casserole dish, preheating the oven before inserting the dish.

First take the chicken from the fridge and allow it to come to room temperature. Then, in a heavy-based frying pan, dry-fry the cumin and fennel seeds over a medium heat for about 2 minutes or until you can smell their heady scent. Remove from the pan and grind into a rough powder using a pestle and mortar or placing in a plastic bag and crushing with a rolling pin. Add the pine nuts to the pan and toast for 3–4 minutes or until golden, shaking the pan regularly to ensure that they don't burn, then set aside to cool.

Finely chop the onion and garlic. Pour the oil into a large saucepan, add the onion and fry over a medium–low heat for 8–10 minutes or until soft and translucent but not browned. Add the garlic and fry for a further couple of minutes, then stir in the freshly ground spices and the quinoa.

Pour over the stock, cover with a lid and bring to the boil, then reduce the heat to low and simmer for 15 minutes or until the quinoa has absorbed all the stock. Finely chop the parsley and dates and stir these into the cooked quinoa with the toasted pine nuts and lemon juice and season well with salt and pepper.

Use half the quinoa mixture to fill the chicken cavity two-thirds full. Place the stuffed bird in the chicken brick or casserole dish and pour 100ml/3½fl oz water into the base. Smear the outside of the chicken with the margarine and season with salt and pepper, then cover with the lid and place in a cold oven (if using the chicken brick).

Turn the oven to 200°C/400°F/gas mark 6 and bake for 1½ hours or until the juices of the chicken run clear when the meat is pierced with a skewer. If using a casserole dish, first preheat the oven and then cook for the same length of time.

Transfer the remaining stuffing to an ovenproof dish and cover with foil. Uncover the chicken and cook for a further 10 minutes to brown, placing the dish of stuffing in the oven at the same time to cook with the chicken. Once the chicken is cooked, leave to rest for 20 minutes in the chicken brick or casserole dish before carving.

Baked Apple and Mustard Ham

Serves 4

—

2kg/4lb 4oz cured
   boneless gammon
2 large sticks of celery
15 juniper berries
5cm/2in cinnamon stick
10 black peppercorns
2 bay leaves
2 litres/3½ pints apple
   juice

For the mustard rub
2 rounded tbsp maple
   syrup
2 tsp mustard powder
1 tbsp demerara sugar

A perfect dish for a winter lunch or supper, the gammon is simmered gently in spiced apple juice and then swathed in a sweet mustard rub before being baked in the oven until the meat is so tender that it simply melts in the mouth. It's delicious served with Parsnip Purée (see page 184) and possibly a roast potato or two. You could eat the leftovers cold with a salad and baked potato or use it to make luxurious sandwiches with my Crusty White Loaf (see page 218). If you wish, you can pre-cook the gammon the night before. Simply simmer it in the apple juice and allow it to cool completely, then cover and store in the fridge. When you are ready to cook, allow it to come up to room temperature and then trim, score and coat with the rub (as below) before baking in the oven, preheated to 180°C/350°F/gas mark 4, for 30–40 minutes.

Place the gammon in a large saucepan – it should be large enough to accommodate the whole piece but still fit snugly. Cover with water and bring to the boil, then drain off the water. Rinse the gammon in cold running water and return it to the saucepan.

Cut the celery into thirds and lightly crush the juniper berries with the back of a wooden spoon, then add these to the pan with the cinnamon stick, peppercorns and bay leaves. Pour over the apple juice, adding a top-up of water if the juice doesn't cover the gammon. Cover with a lid and bring to the boil, then reduce the heat to low and simmer, covering the pan partially with its lid, for 2 hours, checking every now and then that it is still simmering and that all is well.

Preheat the oven to 240°/475°F/gas mark 9.

Carefully lift the gammon out of the apple stock (which you can retain for making risotto or gravy at a later date) and rest on a chopping board, leaving it to cool a little so that you can handle it without burning yourself. Once cooled, cut away the skin, leaving a thin layer of fat. Using a sharp knife, score the fat with diagonal cuts about 2.5cm/1in apart to make large diamond shapes before adding the mustard rub.

Using a wooden spoon or your hands, carefully spread the maple syrup over the skin of the gammon. Sprinkle over the mustard and then the sugar, pressing gently with your hands so that all the ingredients of the rub meld together.

Line a roasting tin with foil, place the gammon on it and then bake in the oven for 10 minutes or until the glaze is caramelised and bubbling. Remove from the oven and leave to rest for 5 minutes before carving into slices to serve.

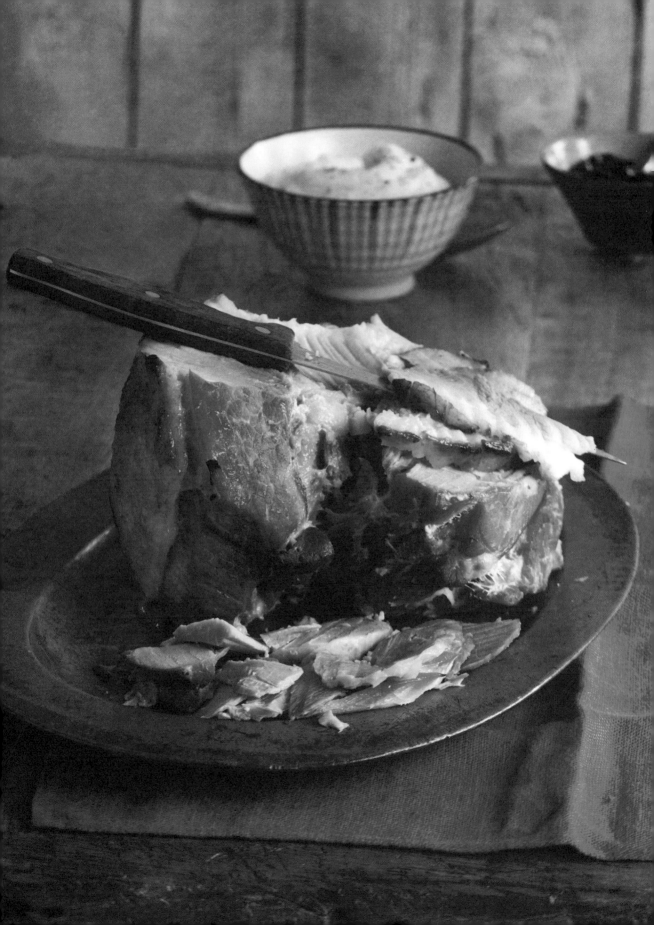

Parsnip Purée

Serves 4–6

—

500g/1lb 2oz parsnips
2 tbsp dairy-free
  margarine (ideally
  Pure Sunflower Spread)
150–200ml/5–7fl oz
  rice milk
Sea salt and freshly
  ground black pepper

Nothing tastes as good on a wintry day than a velvety spoonful of this delicious purée. Divine with my Baked Apple and Mustard Ham (see page 102), it is equally sensational as an accompaniment to roast chicken, lamb cutlets or sausages. I like to steam the parsnips to prevent them becoming watery, while the margarine and rice milk add an ambrosial creaminess to the dish.

Peel and trim the parsnips and cut into 5cm/2in chunks, then place in a steamer or colander set over saucepan containing an inch or two of boiling water (making sure that it doesn't touch the base of the steamer) and steam for around 8 minutes or until completely tender to the point of a knife.

Remove from the pan and tip into a food processor or blender. Add the margarine, pour over the minimum quantity of the rice milk and season well with salt and pepper, then blitz until you have a smooth and creamy purée, adding more rice milk if necessary.

Tip into a saucepan, season further to taste and beat for a final time with a wooden spoon. Serve immediately or heat through when you are ready to serve.

Masala Roast Chicken with Butternut Squash

Serves 4

—

1 large butternut squash

2 red onions

2.5cm/1in piece of root
  ginger

2 cloves of garlic

8 chicken thighs
  (skin left on)

4 tbsp olive oil

1½ tsp garam masala

1 tsp black mustard seeds

1 tsp cumin seeds

A small bunch of coriander

Sea salt and freshly
  ground black pepper

This dish makes a wonderfully warming supper: the marinade of ginger and spices permeates the chicken and butternut squash creating delicious pockets of caramelised spicy crunch when roasted in the oven. You need to prepare this dish a little ahead but the actual cooking, in one pot, couldn't be easier. I recommend serving it with a large bowl of white basmati rice to soak up the gorgeous juices.

Slice the squash in half lengthways and scoop out the seeds and fibres. Peel each half of the squash and then cut into lengths about 2cm/¾in thick. Cut the onions into quarters, peel and grate the ginger and crush the garlic, then place in a sealable plastic bag with the squash, chicken thighs, olive oil and spices. Season well with salt and pepper and leave to marinate in the fridge for between 30 minutes and 3 hours, removing from the fridge 30 minutes before cooking to bring it back up to room temperature.

Preheat the oven to 200°C/400°F/gas mark 6.

Tip the chicken, squash and marinade into a large roasting tin or ovenproof dish and level out evenly. Place in the oven and roast for 40–45 minutes or until cooked through and golden and crispy on top. Remove from the oven and roughly chop the coriander to scatter on top. Serve while hot, being sure to scoop out all the spiced juices and crispy bits from the base of the tin or dish.

Roast Pork Boulangère

Serves 4

—

2 cloves of garlic
3 tsp English mustard
   (3 tsp mustard powder
   mixed with 3 tsp water)
500g/1lb 2oz pork
   tenderloin
3 tsp demerara sugar
4 large floury potatoes
2 eating apples
4 tbsp olive oil
Leaves from a large
   sprig of rosemary
Sea salt and freshly
   ground black pepper

The flavours in this recipe are evocative of northern France – pork tenderloin in a garlicky mustard coating, scented with rosemary and sitting atop a layer of roasted apples and potatoes. This is my favourite kind of dish to cook – ideal come rain or shine and an absolute breeze to prepare.

Preheat the oven to 180°C/350°F/gas mark 4.

Crush the garlic and mix with the mustard, using this to rub all over the outside of the pork. Season well with salt and pepper and sprinkle over the sugar, then leave the pork to rest while you prepare the potatoes and apples.

Peel the potatoes and cut into slices approximately 1cm/½in thick, then peel and halve the apples before cutting into slices of a similar thickness. Pour the olive oil into a large ovenproof dish and then place the apples in the dish and lay the potatoes on top. Season well with salt and pepper and roast in the oven for 45 minutes, shaking the dish every now and then in order to stop the potatoes and apples catching.

Remove from the oven and place the pork on top of the potatoes, scatter over the rosemary leaves and return the dish to the oven, roasting for 25–30 minutes or until the meat is cooked through and tender. Once cooked, remove from the oven and cover in foil. Leave to rest for 10 minutes before slicing and serving.

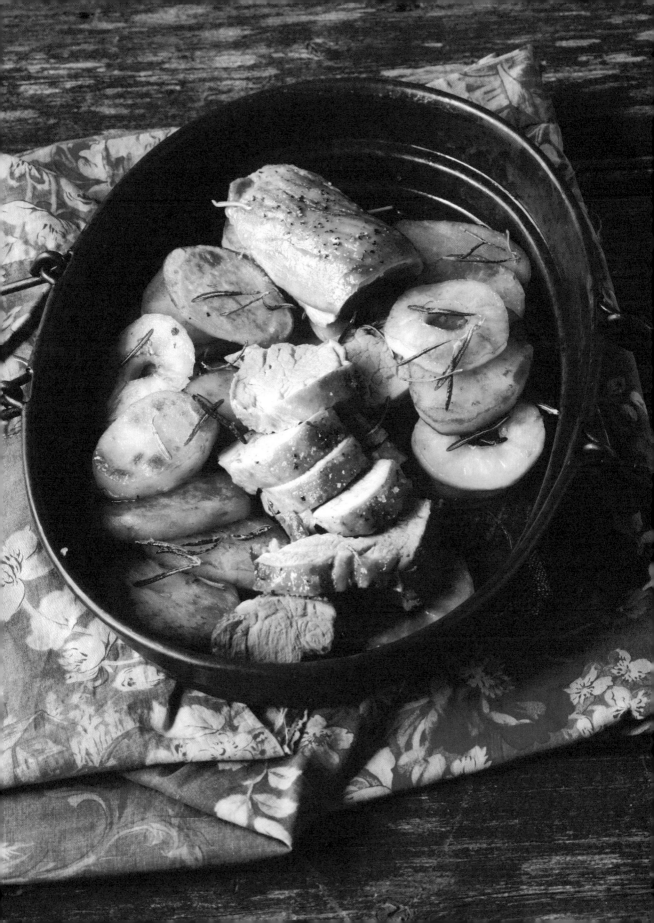

Spicy Sausage and Bean Stew

Serves 4

—

8 gluten-free sausages

2 tbsp olive oil

1 large red onion

2 cloves of garlic

2 tsp soft light brown sugar

1 tsp chilli flakes

¼ tsp smoked paprika

A pinch of ground cinnamon

A pinch of ground cumin

1 x 400g tin of cannellini beans, drained and rinsed

2 x 400g tins of chopped tomatoes

1 tbsp tomato purée

A small bunch of curly-leaf parsley

Juice of ½ lemon

Sea salt and freshly ground black pepper

This is one of those classic dishes that I come back to time and again. When it's cold outside and your day seems to have dragged on longer than it should, this stew will warm the very bottom of your soul. It's a basic, hearty recipe, ideal for preparing for loved ones for an informal supper. Sometimes I serve it with chunks of homemade Crusty White Loaf (see page 218); at others, I spoon it over a bowl of Olive Oil Mashed Potato (see page 192); or I often tip in a handful of kale or spinach to cook through for the final couple of minutes – delicious!

Preheat the oven to 200°C/400°F/gas mark 6.

Lay the sausages in a roasting tin and pour over half the olive oil, then roast in the oven for 25 minutes, turning occasionally to ensure even cooking, until cooked and browned all over. Remove from the oven and set aside.

Finely chop the onion and crush the garlic. Pour the remaining olive oil into a heavy-based saucepan, add the onion and garlic with the sugar and soften over a low heat for about 8 minutes or until almost caramelised.

Add the chilli flakes and ground spices and continue to fry over a low heat for a minute or two. Tip in the beans and warm through, stirring occasionally, and then add the chopped tomatoes and tomato purée.

Finely chop the parsley and slice the cooked sausages into rounds about 2cm/1in thick, then add these and the lemon juice to the tomatoes and beans and season well with salt and pepper. Cover the saucepan with a lid, then bring to the boil, reduce the heat to low and cook for 30 minutes so that the flavours can really develop before serving. Alternatively, reduce the oven temperature to 180°C/350°F/gas mark 4 and cook the stew in a casserole dish or ovenproof saucepan for the same length of time.

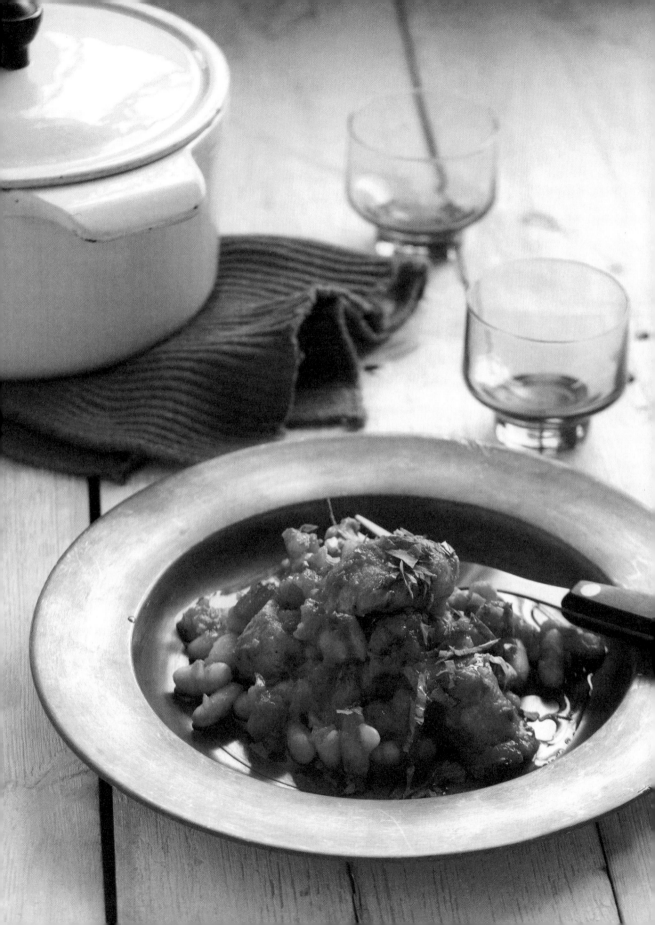

Pasta with Smoky Bacon, Olive and Chilli Tomato Sauce

Serves 4

—

4 plum tomatoes or
    1 x 400g tin of plum
    tomatoes
100g/3½oz pitted
    black olives
1 red onion
6 rashers of smoked
    streaky bacon
1 tbsp olive oil
1 tsp chilli flakes
1 tsp soft light brown
    sugar
1 x 700g jar of passata
2 tsp tomato purée
A small bunch of
    curly-leaf parsley
400g/14oz gluten-free
    tricolore fusilli or other
    pasta of your choice
Sea salt and freshly
    ground black pepper

This is a delightful dish to tuck into on a wintry evening. I often make double the quantity of sauce and freeze the extra so that I always have some to hand. A range of gluten-free pasta is available in most supermarkets, including a number of very good-quality brands. They cook just as well as 'real' pasta and I defy most people to be able to tell the difference between the two. See Products and Stockists on page 232 for details.

First skin the fresh plum tomatoes (if using) by placing them in a bowl, covering in boiling water and leaving for 1 minute. Drain and carefully peel away the tomato skins (they should slide off with ease), then slice in half, scoop out the seeds and chop the flesh into 1cm/½in pieces. If using tinned plum tomatoes, drain away the excess juice and then chop into 1cm/½in chunks.

Slice the olives into small rounds, finely dice the onion and chop the bacon into 2cm/¾in pieces. Pour the olive oil into a large, heavy-based saucepan and fry the bacon over a medium–high heat for 3–4 minutes or until crispy and golden. Using a slotted spoon, remove the bacon from the pan and set aside.

Using the same pan, lower the heat and gently fry the diced onion in the remaining bacon fat for 2–3 minutes or until softened. Add the chilli flakes, diced tomatoes and sugar, season with salt and pepper and stir all the ingredients together.

Add the passata and tomato purée to the pan, then finely chop the parsley and add to the sauce with the olives, seasoning further to taste. Cover with a lid and bring to the boil, then reduce the heat to low and simmer gently for 30 minutes.

Meanwhile, bring a large saucepan of salted water to the boil, add the pasta and cook until al dente following the instructions on the packet – usually 10–12 minutes, depending on the brand. Drain the pasta and add to the sauce, stirring in gently and heating through before serving.

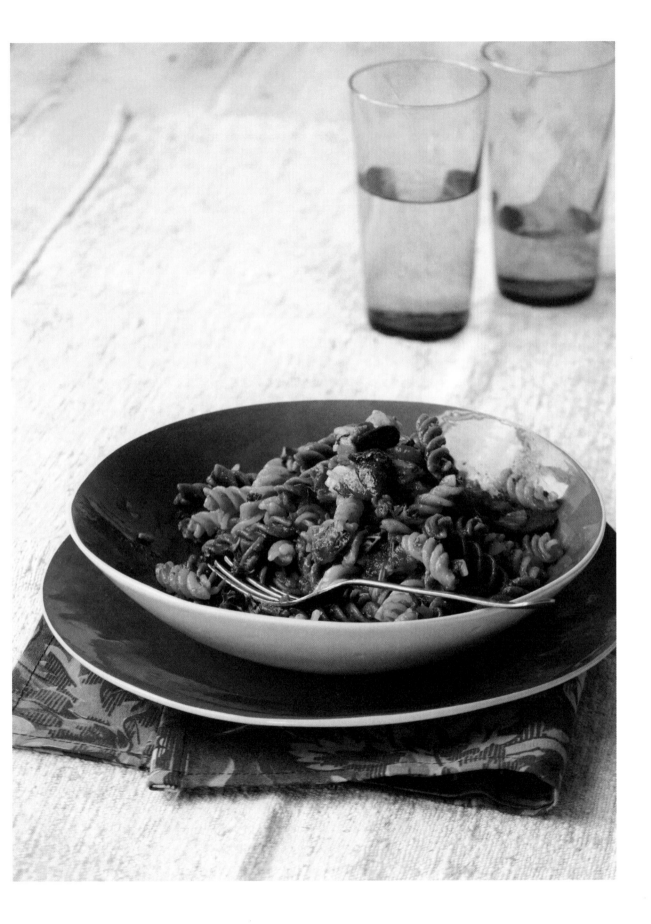

Roast Beef with Horseradish Cream and Olive Oil Mashed Potato

Serves 4

—

1.25kg/2lb 12oz beef
  sirloin or rib of beef
2 large cloves of garlic
1 tsp mustard powder
Sea salt and freshly
  ground black pepper

For the mashed potatoes
450g/1lb floury potatoes
  (such as Maris Piper)
4 tbsp extra-virgin
  olive oil
Sea salt and freshly
  ground black pepper

For the horseradish cream
75g/3oz fresh horseradish
150ml/5fl oz oat cream
Juice of ¼ lemon
Sea salt and freshly
  ground black pepper

A truly English institution, roast beef and horseradish cream are a wonderful treat to serve on a cold winter's day. I like to accompany mine with these mashed potatoes and a bowl of honey-roasted carrots, but any seasonal vegetables would do just as well. To achieve the best results, I advocate roasting beef in the way I've done here: that is, cooking it for 20 minutes in a hot oven, in order to brown it, before lowering the heat and cooking for a further 20 minutes per 450g/1lb for medium or 10 minutes per 450g/1lb for rare. Whatever the size of your joint, always allow 20 minutes' resting time before serving – the meat will be so much more tender and you will really taste the difference.

Preheat the oven to 220°C/425°F/gas mark 7 and remove the beef from the fridge to bring it up to room temperature.

Cut the garlic cloves in half lengthways. Using a small, sharp knife and cutting to a depth of about 1cm/½in, pierce four equally spaced holes in the beef and insert one shard of garlic into each hole. Sprinkle the mustard powder over the beef and season well with salt and pepper, then place in a roasting tin and roast in the oven for 20 minutes.

Meanwhile, peel and finely grate the horseradish. Mix with the oat cream and lemon juice and season well with salt and pepper, then cover and leave in the fridge until the beef is cooked. (The cream will thicken up once it is chilled.)

After you have roasted the beef for 20 minutes, lower the temperature of the oven to 160°C/325°F/gas mark 3 and continue to cook for a further 30 minutes for rare or 55 minutes for medium. Remove from the oven, cover with foil and leave to rest for 20 minutes before carving.

While the beef is resting, peel and cut the potatoes into 2.5cm/1in cubes. Place in a large saucepan of salted water (the water should cover the potatoes by a couple of centimetres) and bring to the boil. Once boiling, reduce the heat and simmer for about 15 minutes or until completely cooked through and soft to the point of a knife. Drain the potatoes and return to the pan, adding the olive oil and seasoning with salt and pepper. Mash until smooth and creamy and then serve with the carved roast beef and horseradish cream.

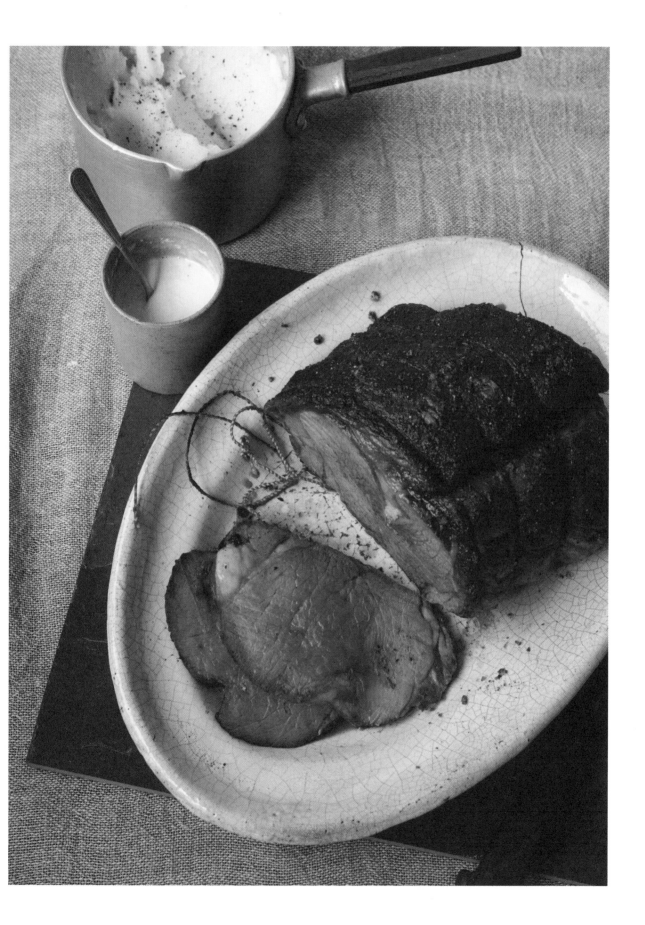

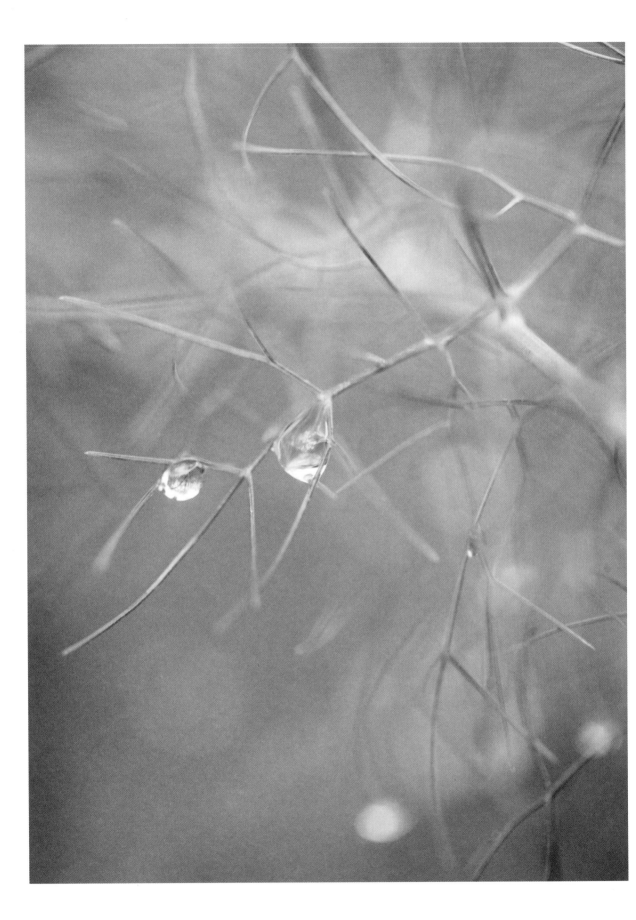

Spiced Lamb Steaks with Chickpea Purée

Serves 4

—

4 lamb steaks, about
  2cm/¾in thick
2 tbsp hot water
2 tbsp runny honey
1 tsp allergy-friendly
  stock powder
2 cloves of garlic
A small bunch of mint
1 tsp chilli flakes
1 tsp ground cumin

For the chickpea purée
1 white onion
2 cloves of garlic
2 x 400g tins of chickpeas,
  drained and rinsed
600ml/1 pint vegetable
  stock
1½ tbsp olive oil
Sea salt and freshly
  ground black pepper

Lamb is such a rich meat that it can really hold its own with other strong flavours. Here, the spicy marinade imbues the lamb steaks, intensifying in flavour when seared in the griddle pan. The chickpea purée really complements this dish, as it would virtually any roasted meat or stew. With its light and creamy texture, it makes a fantastic alternative to mashed potato.

Trim any excess fat from the lamb steaks and place in a shallow dish, then mix together the hot water, honey and stock powder in a separate bowl and stir until the stock powder has dissolved. Crush the garlic and finely chop the mint and add to the marinade with the chilli flakes and cumin, stirring to combine. Pour over the lamb steaks, cover and leave to marinate for around 2 hours.

Meanwhile, make the chickpea purée. Finely chop the onion and garlic and tip into a saucepan with the chickpeas, then pour in the vegetable stock and enough water so that the chickpeas are just covered. Bring to the boil, then reduce the heat to low and simmer for 15 minutes.

Next add the olive oil to a heavy-based saucepan and sauté the onions and garlic over a medium heat for around 8 minutes or until soft but not browned. Drain the cooked chickpeas, reserving all the liquid. Place the chickpeas and onion in a food processor, season well with salt and pepper and blitz, adding the reserved stock bit by bit, until you have a smooth purée. (You may not need to add all the stock.) Return to the saucepan, season further to taste and reheat when you are ready to serve.

Heat a griddle pan or heavy-based frying pan until very hot and sear the lamb steaks for about 6 minutes on each side, basting with the marinade as you go. Set aside to rest for 5–10 minutes and then serve with the chickpea purée.

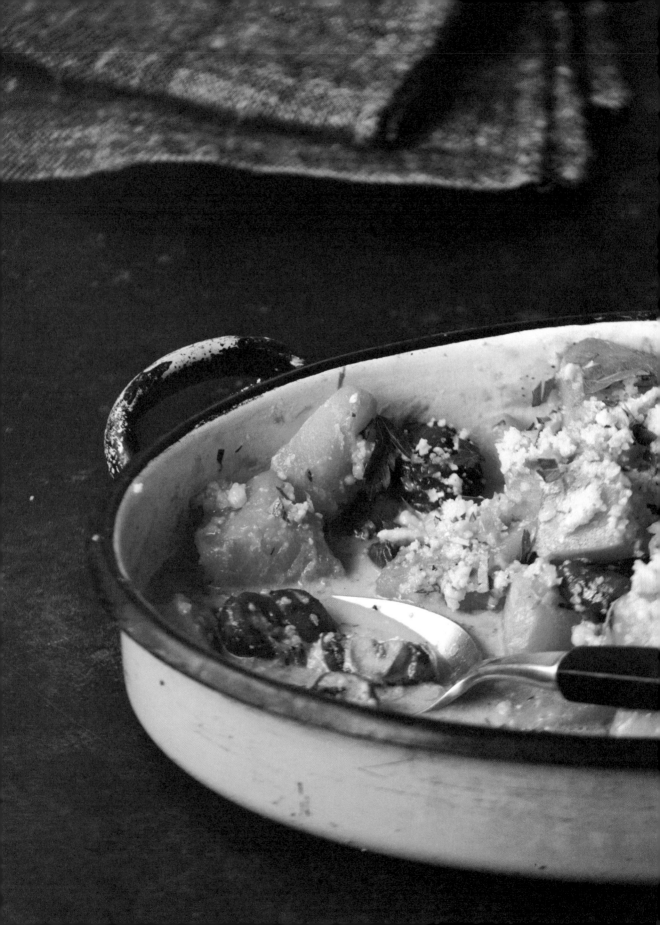

Winter Squash and Chestnut Bake

Serves 4
Contains nuts
—
100g/3½oz pine nuts
1 butternut squash
1 onion
3 cloves of garlic
250g/9oz chestnut
   mushrooms
200g/7oz cooked
   and peeled chestnuts
50g/1¾oz dairy-free
   margarine (ideally
   Pure Sunflower Spread)
½ tbsp olive oil
Leaves from 6 sprigs
   of thyme
250ml/9fl oz oat cream
A small bunch of
   curly-leaf parsley
Sea salt and freshly
   ground black pepper

There is something truly satisfying about this combination of baked mushrooms, chestnuts and butternut squash, with its rich woodland taste and meaty texture. The oat cream and ground pine nuts produce a rich, creamy sauce, while the garlic and thyme – both firm friends of the mushroom and chestnut – permeate the dish with a rounded intensity of flavour.

In a heavy-based frying pan, dry-fry the pine nuts over a medium–high heat for 3–4 minutes or until golden, shaking the pan regularly to ensure that they don't burn. Remove from the heat and allow to cool. Then, using a food processor, grind the pine nuts until they are of a fine, breadcrumb-like consistency.

Slice the butternut squash in half and scoop out the seeds and fibres, then peel the squash halves and cut into 2.5cm/1in chunks. Finely dice the onion and garlic and cut the mushrooms into halves or quarters, depending on their size.

Heat the margarine and olive oil in a large, heavy-based saucepan until the margarine is foaming (the addition of the olive oil will stop it burning). Add the garlic, onion and thyme and season well with salt and pepper, then sauté over a low heat for about 10 minutes or until the onion becomes soft but not browned.

Add the butternut squash to the pan, turn the heat up slightly and cook, stirring occasionally, for 5 minutes or until the pieces of squash start to give when pressed. Add the mushrooms, mix in thoroughly and cook for a further 5 minutes or until both mushrooms and squash are tender.

Preheat the oven to 200°C/400°F/gas mark 6.

Next add the oat cream and chestnuts to the pan and season liberally with salt and pepper. Bring the dish to the boil, then reduce the heat to low and simmer for 5 minutes. Spoon the squash and mushroom mixture into an ovenproof dish and sprinkle evenly with the ground, toasted pine nuts. Bake in the oven for 10–15 minutes or until the dish is bubbling and golden on top, then finely chop the parsley and sprinkle over to serve.

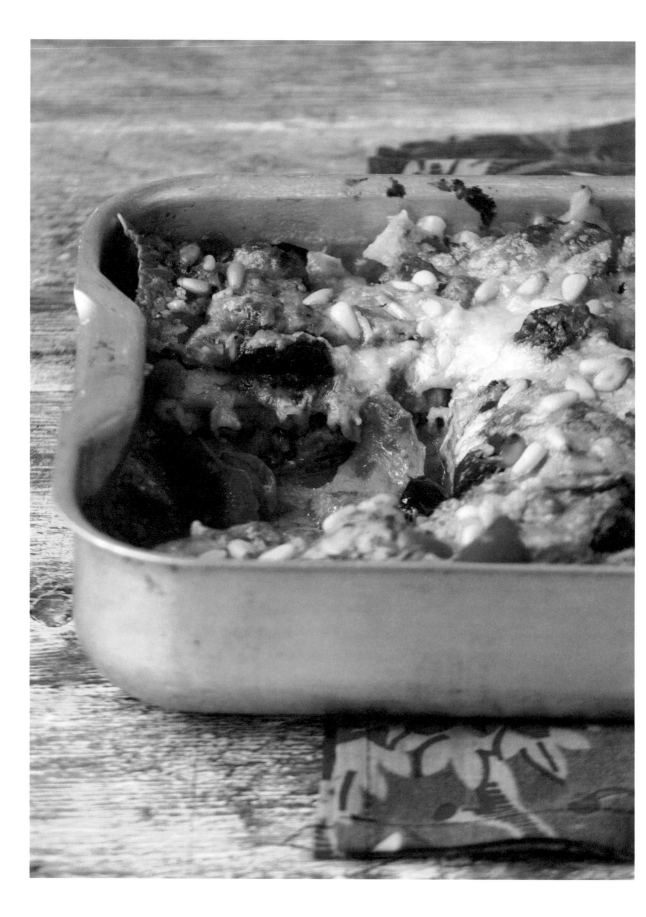

Vegetable Lasagne

Serves 4
Contains nuts
—

1 yellow pepper
1 red pepper
1 aubergine
1 red onion
2 courgettes
2 cloves of garlic
2 tbsp olive oil
500ml/18fl oz passata
140g/5oz sun-blushed
  tomatoes
1 tsp soft light brown
  sugar
2 tsp lemon juice
A small bunch of oregano
A large bunch of basil
6 large or 12 small sheets
  of gluten- and egg-free
  lasagne
Sea salt and freshly
  ground black pepper

For the white sauce
150g/5oz pine nuts, plus
  extra for scattering
300ml/½ pint rice milk
300ml/½ pint vegetable
  stock
50g/2oz Pure Sunflower
  Spread (dairy-free
  margarine)
50g/2oz gluten-free plain
  flour (ideally Doves Farm)
Sea salt and freshly
  ground black pepper

You will need a 25 x 19cm/
7 x 10in ovenproof dish for
this recipe

This is a delicious vegetarian dish that really proves that intolerance-friendly food can taste amazing. I love the simplicity of the white sauce, made rich with the flavour of ground, toasted pine nuts. It is important to note that the natural oil content of pine nuts can vary from batch to batch, so you may find that sometimes they pull together in a roux and at others they remain dry and crumbly. This can affect the consistency of the sauce so whisking the ingredients together well is key to its success. If the sauce looks as if it is splitting, don't panic; just lower the heat and continue to whisk vigorously until it pulls back together.

Preheat the oven to 200°C/400°F/gas mark 6.

Deseed the peppers and cut these, the aubergine and the onion into 2cm/¾in chunks. Halve the courgettes lengthways and cut into half-moons 1cm/½in thick. Crush the garlic and combine with all the prepared vegetables in a large roasting tin. Add the olive oil and mix together thoroughly, then roast in the oven for 35 minutes, stirring every now and then.

While the vegetables are cooking, prepare the pine nuts for the white sauce. Scatter the pine nuts on a baking tray and toast in the oven, turning them occasionally to make sure they don't burn, for 8–10 minutes or until golden brown, then remove and set aside to cool. Once cooled, place in a food processor and pulse until they are of a fine-breadcrumb consistency.

In a large saucepan, combine the passata with the sun-blushed tomatoes, sugar and lemon juice. Finely chop the oregano and basil, adding these to the pan, then stir in the roasted vegetables and season with salt and pepper.

Next make the white sauce. Pour the milk and stock into a saucepan and heat gently until warm but not simmering. Melt the margarine in another saucepan over a low heat, add the flour and stir vigorously with a wooden spoon for 1 minute to form a thick roux. Cook for 30 seconds, stirring continuously, then add the ground, toasted pine nuts and stir into the roux until fully combined. Remove from the heat, pour in the hot milk and stock in stages and whisk it into the roux bit by bit, returning it to a low heat, until the sauce is smooth, thick and creamy. Season with salt and pepper to taste and set aside.

To make up the lasagne, pour a small amount of the vegetable mixture into the base of the ovenproof dish, spreading it out evenly with

recipe continues >

> *continued from previous page*

the back of a spoon. Cover with half the sheets of lasagne (three large or six small sheets) add a further thin layer of vegetable mixture. Pour over half the white sauce, spreading it out in an even layer, then lay the remaining lasagne sheets over the top, cover with the remaining vegetable sauce and pour over the final layer of white sauce.

Sprinkle over some whole pine nuts, cover loosely with foil and bake in the oven for 40 minutes. After 25 minutes, remove the foil and bake until golden and bubbling.

Peppers stuffed with Gado Gado Sauce

Serves 4
Contains nuts
—

4 peppers (red, yellow or orange)
A small bunch of coriander

For the sauce
2 cloves of garlic
1 red onion
1 red chilli
2.5cm/1in piece of root ginger
2 tbsp olive oil
3 tbsp crunchy peanut butter
1 x 400g tin of chopped tomatoes
1 tbsp tomato purée
Sea salt and freshly ground black pepper

I can't tell you how delicious this sauce is: it has a real punch of flavour that makes for an exciting, nutty, spiced dish. I have used it here as a filling for roasted peppers, but it works just as well poured over roasted vegetables (parsnips, carrots and cauliflower spring to mind) or baked squash. The sweetness of the vegetables and the spicy richness of the sauce go so well together, especially when accompanied by a big bowl of brown rice. I urge you to experiment with different combinations to find your favourite one.

Cut each pepper in half lengthways, slicing through the stalk so that each half has part of its stalk left attached. Carefully remove the seeds and white pith from each pepper half, cutting around the stalk, and set aside.

Next make the sauce. Finely chop the garlic and onion, deseed and finely chop the chilli and peel and grate the ginger. Add the olive oil to a heavy-based saucepan and fry the onion, garlic, chilli and ginger over a low–medium heat for about 6 minutes or until the onion is soft but not browned. Add the peanut butter, tomatoes and tomato purée to the pan, season with salt and pepper. Cover with a lid and cook over a low heat for 30 minutes, stirring occasionally.

Meanwhile, preheat the oven to 200°C/400°F/gas mark 6.

Place the pepper halves on a baking tray. Fill each half with the spicy peanut sauce, cover loosely in foil and bake in the oven for 50 minutes. Finely chop the coriander and sprinkle over the cooked peppers to serve.

Spiced Parsnip Quinoa

Serves 4
Contains nuts

—

1 tbsp runny honey
2 tbsp groundnut oil
1 tsp smoked paprika
1 tsp ground cumin
500g/1lb 2oz parsnips
40g/1½oz pine nuts
175g/6oz quinoa
500ml/18fl oz vegetable
   stock
A bunch of coriander
Sea salt and freshly
   ground black pepper

This is a real fire-in-your-belly kind of meal, injecting warmth and energy and bursting with flavour. The parsnips are slow-baked in cumin, paprika and honey and combined with light and fluffy quinoa, golden toasted pine nuts and fresh, tangy coriander. I love to make this for a winter lunch and nearly always serve it with a good dollop of houmous and a large green salad dressed in lemon juice and olive oil.

Preheat the oven to 200°C/400°F/gas mark 6.

Add the honey to a large bowl and combine with the groundnut oil, paprika, cumin and 1 teaspoon of salt. Peel and trim the parsnips, cutting them into batons approximately 5cm/2in long and 1cm/½in thick. Add these to the bowl and mix thoroughly to ensure they are well coated in the marinade, then leave to marinate for 30 minutes.

Pour the parsnips and marinade into a non-stick roasting tin, cover tightly with foil and bake in the oven for 45 minutes, turning every now and then to ensure that they don't stick. Take out of the oven, remove the foil and then return to cook for a further 10 minutes or until the parsnips are beginning to caramelise on the outside.

Meanwhile, scatter the pine nuts on a baking tray and toast in the oven, turning them occasionally to make sure they don't burn, for 5–6 minutes or until golden brown, then remove and set aside to cool.

Shortly before the parsnips have finished cooking, place the quinoa in a saucepan and pour over the stock, then cover with a lid and bring to the boil. Once boiling, reduce the heat to low and leave to simmer very gently for approximately 15 minutes or until all of the stock has been absorbed by the quinoa.

Using a fork, gently fluff up the cooked quinoa, season well with salt and pepper and combine in a large serving bowl with the roasted parsnips and pine nuts. Finely chop the coriander and mix in, then serve while warm.

Chocolate and Chestnut Cake

Serves 8
Contains nuts

—

110g/4oz Pure Sunflower
 Spread (dairy-free
 margarine), plus extra
 for greasing
4 tbsp ground flaxseeds
1¾ tsp baking powder
150g/5oz crème de
 marrons (sweetened
 chestnut purée)
110g/4oz gluten-free plain
 flour (ideally Doves Farm)
2 tbsp cocoa powder
A very small pinch of
 sea salt
6 tbsp rice milk

For the ganache
75g/3oz dairy-free
 dark chocolate
100g/3½oz crème
 de marrons

You will need a 20cm/
8in diameter cake tin
with a removable base
for this recipe

This is a truly irresistible cake; although perhaps calling it a cake is a little misleading. It has a thin sponge base, only a finger-width deep, with a rich ganache topping made from a mixture of melted chocolate and crème de marrons – a sweetened chestnut purée. Highly versatile, this purée can be made into ice cream or a patisserie filling, among other delicious things. Used here, it gives this cake a wonderfully velvety texture, simply oozing with decadence.

Preheat the oven to 170°C/325°F/gas mark 3, then lightly grease the cake tin and line the base with baking parchment.

Make up the egg replacer mixture by blending the ground flaxseeds with ¼ teaspoon of the baking powder and 6 tablespoons of water, then set aside for a few minutes. The flax will swell up and absorb the water so that you are left with a thick paste rather than a liquid.

Next, in a large bowl stir together the margarine and chestnut purée gently with a wooden spoon until pale, light and fluffy. Add the egg replacer mixture, a little at a time and whisking as you go, until fully incorporated into the purée. Sift in the flour with the cocoa powder, salt and remaining baking powder, then fold into the purée using a large metal spoon. Pour in the rice milk and continue to fold all the ingredients together until fully combined.

Spoon the cake mixture into the prepared tin, levelling the top with the back of your spoon, and bake in the oven for 35 minutes or until risen and springy to a light touch, then remove from the oven and transfer to a wire rack to cool.

Meanwhile, place a heatproof bowl over a small saucepan containing 2.5cm/1in of simmering water. Break up the chocolate into the bowl and melt, stirring occasionally, until smooth and glossy, then remove from the heat and stir in the chestnut purée. When the cake has cooled, spread over the chocolate and chestnut ganache and cut into slices to serve.

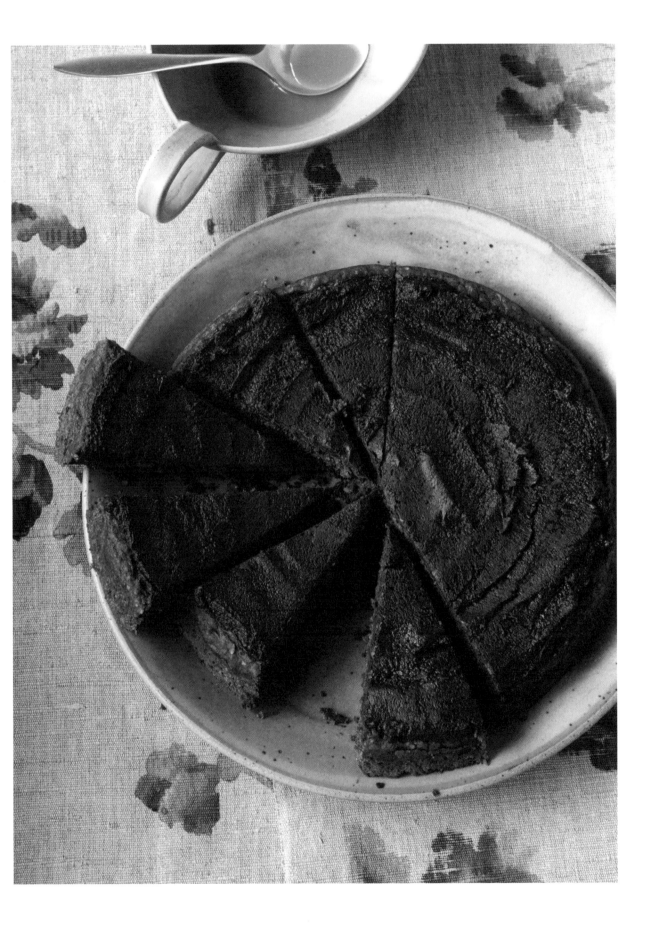

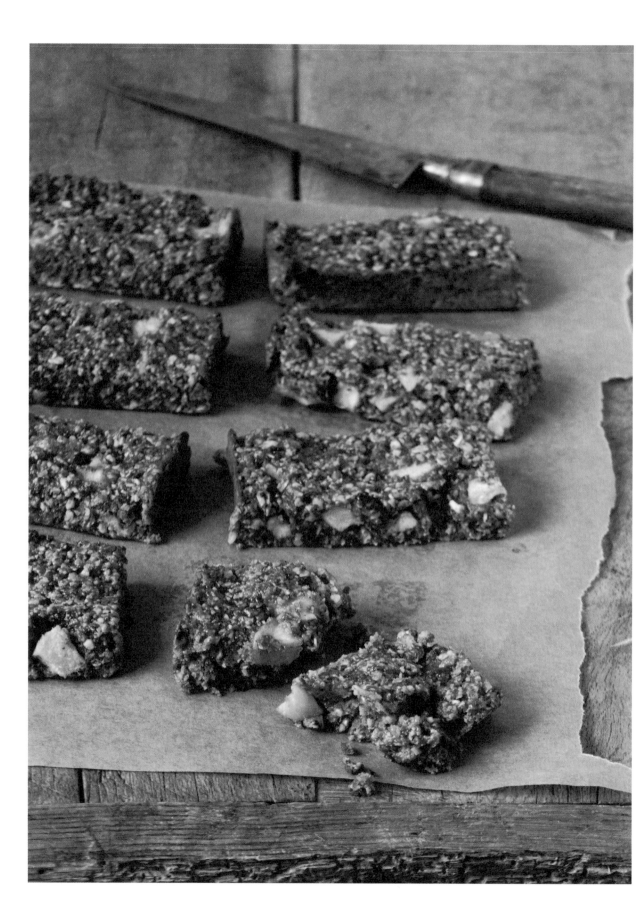

Apple and Cinnamon Granola Bars

Serves 8
Contains nuts
—

100g/3½oz jumbo
    porridge oats
240g/8½oz mixed dried
    fruit and nuts (such as
    apricots, raisins, dates,
    almonds, walnuts and
    pecans)
2 tbsp ground flaxseeds
2 tbsp smooth peanut
    or almond butter
150ml/5fl oz agave syrup

For the apple pieces
1 large eating apple
1 tbsp lemon juice
1 tbsp agave syrup
¼ tsp ground cinnamon

*You will need a 20cm/8in
square baking tin for this
recipe*

*Apple and cinnamon seem to have been made for each other, and I just
adore these bars, in which the fruit and spice are combined in a divinely
nutty mixture. Baking apple pieces in this way retains their sweetness and
gives them a pleasantly chewy texture. I quite often make a large quantity
of them to sprinkle on cereal or porridge for breakfast, or to add to Vanilla
Ice Cream (see page 66) for a quick pudding. If you would like to make
extra, just adjust the quantities accordingly – six eating apples combined
with 1 teaspoon of ground cinnamon and 4 tablespoons each of lemon
juice and agave syrup. Once cooked, these granola bars will keep in an
airtight container in the fridge for up to a week.*

Preheat the oven to 170°C/325°F/gas mark 3, then line a baking tray
with baking parchment.

Prepare the apples by peeling and coring them, then chop into
5mm/¼in cubes and place in a bowl. Add the lemon juice, agave syrup
and cinnamon and stir together so that the apple pieces are coated in the
syrup mixture. Spread the apple pieces over the parchment in an even
layer and bake in the oven for 25 minutes, then remove and set aside.

Increase the oven temperature to 180°C/350°F/gas mark 4.

Next, combine all the remaining ingredients in a food processor and
pulse until finely chopped, and then continue to pulse until the mixture
pulls together. Transfer the mixture to a bowl and fold in the cooked
apple pieces.

Tip the granola mixture into the prepared baking tray and, using a
spatula, spread and push the mixture into the sides of the tray, smoothing
the surface so that it is level and even. Bake in the oven for 15 minutes,
then remove and use a sharp knife to divide the mixture into eight bars.
Return to the oven for a further 10 minutes or until golden. Once
cooked, leave in the baking tray to cool completely before cutting out
the bars and removing from the tray.

Little Sticky Toffee Puddings

Serves 6

—

50g/1¾oz Pure
   Sunflower Spread,
   plus extra for greasing
175g/6oz pitted dates
1 tsp bicarbonate of soda
300ml/½ pint boiling
   water
175g/6oz caster sugar
2 heaped tsp egg replacer
   (ideally Orgran) whisked
   with 4 tbsp of water
175g/6oz gluten-free
   self-raising flour
   (ideally Doves Farm)
½ tsp xanthan gum
½ tsp vanilla extract

For the toffee sauce
100g/3½oz Pure
   Sunflower Spread
   (dairy-free margarine)
150g/5½oz soft light
   brown sugar
125ml/4½fl oz oat cream

*You will need six 8cm/
3in diameter pudding
tins, with a depth of about
5cm/2in, for this recipe*

Nothing, I repeat, nothing symbolises the warm embrace of winter comfort more than a sticky toffee pudding. There are a host of delicious sweet, baked goods to be had, but these puddings put most of them in the shade. This particular recipe is right up there with the best and a feat of allergen-free engineering – even if I say so myself!

Preheat the oven to 180°C/350°F/gas mark 4 and lightly grease the pudding tins.

Chop the dates into small pieces and place in a bowl. Mix in the bicarbonate of soda, pour over the boiling water and leave to stand.

In a large bowl, cream together the margarine and sugar gently with a wooden spoon and then pour in the egg replacer mixture, adding a little at a time and beating well between each addition. Sift in the flour and xanthan gum and gently fold in, then stir in the date mixture (liquid and all) and vanilla extract until fully amalgamated and forming a thick batter.

Pour into the individual tins (the mixture should come to just under the rim of each mould), place on a baking tray and bake in the centre of the oven for 25–30 minutes or until cooked through – a cocktail stick inserted into the centre of each pudding should come out clean.

While the puddings are cooking, make the toffee sauce. Melt the margarine with the sugar in a small saucepan, stirring continuously over a medium heat until smooth and glossy. Pour in the oat cream and bring to a very gentle simmer, then heat the mixture through for 5 minutes, stirring every now and then to ensure the oat cream doesn't curdle.

Once the puddings are cooked, remove from the oven and leave for a few minutes in their tins. Run a sharp knife around the outside edge of each pudding to help loosen it in the mould and carefully tip out onto a serving plate. Pour a portion of the toffee sauce over the pudding and serve while hot.

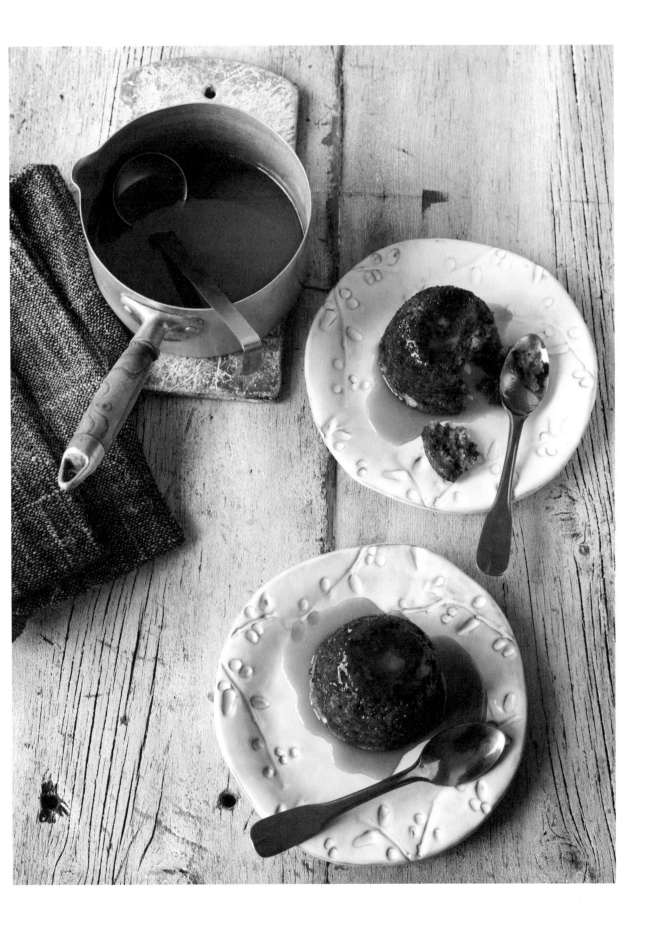

Treacle Tart with Custard

Serves 8
Contains nuts

—

1 quantity of sweet
  Shortcrust Pastry
  (see page 223)

For the filling
75g/3oz gluten-free
  cornflakes
300g/11oz golden syrup
Grated zest and juice of
  ½ lemon

For the custard
2 tbsp golden caster sugar
½ tsp vanilla paste
3 tbsp dairy- and gluten-
  free custard powder
500ml/18fl oz rice milk
4 tsp cornflour

*You will need a 23cm/
9in diameter tart tin
with a removable base
for this recipe*

Oh, the delights of warm treacle tart on a chilly winter's day – there really is no other season of the year to which it seems so well suited. For this particular version of the dish I've borrowed an old trick from the Women's Institute – using cornflakes in place of breadcrumbs. The result is a delectably gooey tart, perfect for serving with lashings of allergy-friendly hot custard.

Preheat the oven to 190°C/375°F/gas mark 5.

Roll out the pastry and fill the tart tin following the instructions given in the Shortcrust Pastry recipe on page 223.

Next make the filling. Crush the cornflakes in a food processor or by placing them in a plastic bag and bashing with a rolling pin. Melt the golden syrup in a saucepan over a low heat, then tip in the crushed cornflakes, add the lemon zest and juice and stir together. Pour the filling into the tart case and bake in the oven for 30–35 minutes or until just set. Transfer the tin to a cooling rack and leave for a few minutes before cutting the tart into slices.

To make the custard, mix together the sugar, vanilla paste and custard powder with a dash of rice milk to form a smooth paste. Pour in the remaining milk and whisk together, then pour into a small saucepan, add the cornflour and cook over a medium heat, whisking continuously, for 3–4 minutes or until thickened and smooth. Pour over each slice of treacle tart and serve while hot.

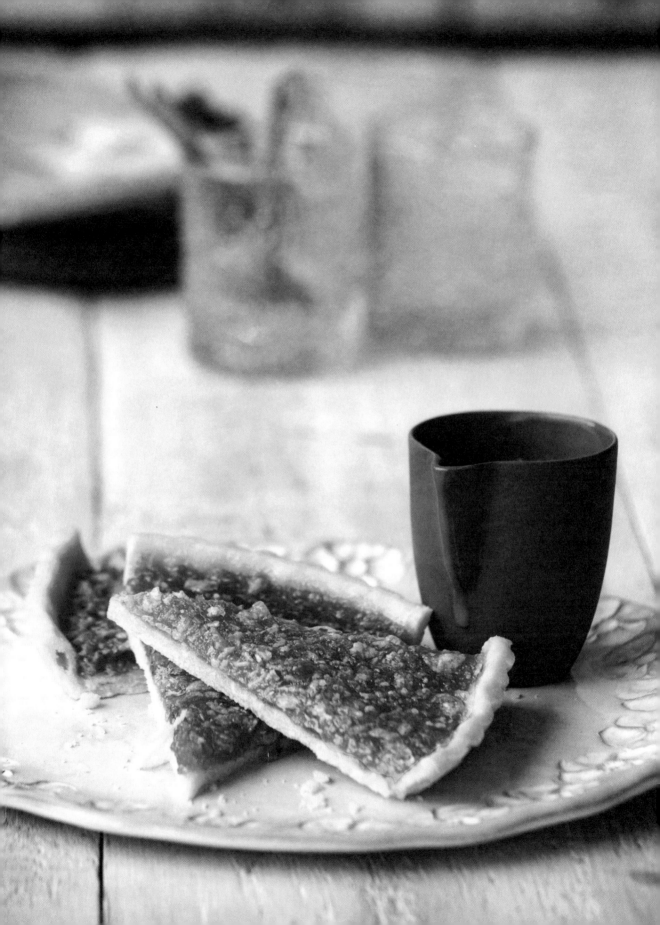

Lemon, Sesame and Ginger Cake

Serves 8

—

100g/3½oz Pure
    Sunflower Spread
    (dairy-free margarine),
    plus extra for greasing
125g/4½oz gluten-free
    self-raising flour
    (ideally Doves Farm)
1 tbsp sesame seeds
2 heaped tsp egg replacer
    (ideally Orgran) whisked
    with 4 tbsp water
125g/4½oz golden caster
    sugar
Grated zest and juice
    of 1 lemon
1 tsp ground ginger

For the icing
1 ball of stem ginger
100g/3½oz icing sugar
1–2 tbsp warm water

*You will need a 900g/2lb
loaf tin for this recipe*

Baking is a joy that should be denied to no one, especially those with food sensitivities. Taking the time to bake a cake can bring as much pleasure as the act of eating it; just as offering it to others is a way of showing that you care. This is a lovely, lightly spiced cake with the warmth of ginger, brightness of lemon and a mellow background note of sesame. Enjoy baking and sharing it with friends and family, or indulging in a slice for yourself with a cup of tea.

Preheat the oven to 170°C/325°F/gas mark 3, then lightly grease the loaf tin and line the base and sides with baking parchment.

Sift the flour into a large bowl and add the sesame seeds, stirring together to combine. (This will stop the sesame seeds from sinking to the bottom of the cake.) Add the egg replacer mixture and all the remaining ingredients and beat together until smooth and glossy.

Spoon the cake batter into the prepared loaf tin, levelling the top with the back of your spoon, and bake in the oven for 45 minutes or until slightly risen and a skewer inserted into the centre of the cake comes out clean. Remove from the oven and allow to cool in the tin for a minute or two before turning out onto a wire rack and leaving to cool down completely while you make the icing.

Finely chop the ginger and add to a bowl. Sift in the icing sugar and add 1 tablespoon of the warm water, mixing everything together until smooth and glossy. Add the remaining water, bit by bit, if you think the icing needs it – you want it to be spreadable yet thick enough to coat the back of a spoon. Once the cake is completely cool, spread over the icing and cut the cake into slices to serve.

Maple and Pecan Squares

Makes 20 squares
Contains nuts

—

150g/5oz Pure Sunflower
  Spread (dairy-free
  margarine), plus extra
  for greasing
125g/4½oz soft dark
  brown sugar
250ml/9fl oz maple syrup
1 tsp vanilla extract
2 tsp mixed spice
2 heaped tsp egg replacer
  (ideally Orgran) whisked
  with 4 tbsp water
1 tsp bicarbonate of soda
  mixed with 2 tbsp
  warm water
300g/11oz gluten-free
  plain flour (ideally
  Doves Farm)
100g/3½oz pecan nuts

*You will need a 20 x 30cm/
8 x 10in ovenproof dish or
roasting tin for this recipe*

*For me the words 'maple' and 'pecan' conjure up charm and comfort, as
homely and reassuring as a quilted blanket or a freshly brewed cup of tea.
These squares are mellow-tasting and light-textured, the pecans giving a
nice nutty bite. They're a pleasure to make and breathing in their fabulous
aroma as they cook is almost as good as eating them. You could serve the
squares dusted in icing sugar or covered in an orange or lemon icing (see
page 112), but they're also delicious just as they are.*

Preheat the oven to 170°C/325°F/gas mark 3, then lightly grease the
ovenproof dish or roasting tin and line the base and sides with baking
parchment.

Place the margarine in a saucepan over a low heat and add the sugar,
maple syrup, vanilla extract and mixed spice. Heat gently, stirring
occasionally, until the margarine has melted and combined with the
sugar and syrup. Remove from the heat, leave to cool for a minute and
then add the egg replacer and bicarbonate of soda mixture.

Sift the flour into a large bowl, break the pecans into small pieces
and mix with the flour. Pour in the liquid ingredients and whisk together
until the batter is smooth (except for the nuts) and glossy.

Pour the mixture into the lined dish or tin (you needn't worry about
levelling the batter as it is so runny) and bake in the oven for 45 minutes
or until risen and springy to a light touch. Transfer the dish or tin to a
wire rack and allow the cake to cool before cutting into squares.

Breads and Baking

Breads and baking are often the trickiest aspects of cooking allergy-friendly food. In my experience, cooking in an allergy-free way sometimes means having to forget what you've previously known about baking methods. Basic principles that would work for a dish containing gluten or eggs may no longer apply to its allergy-friendly alternative. Each recipe in this book contains clear and easy-to-use instructions, but before you begin let me offer you a few tips that have always helped me.

Traditionally, the method of kneading bread vigorously helps to release the gluten in the wheat flour. Because the flour used in this book is gluten free, there is no need to be so rough with the dough. In fact, over kneading can damage the bread, as it squeezes out any air that has been incorporated and stops it from rising, albeit only slightly! When kneading is called for in a recipe, only a light touch is required and for a short amount of time. Simply balling and lightly stretching the dough – which helps the xanthan gum release its elasticity – is all that is needed. Don't be tempted to treat it too roughly.

Shortcrust pastry dough usually needs to be chilled and then blind baked in a hot oven. However, my shortcrust pastry needs none of this, which makes it a lot easier to use than its classic counterpart. Once you have made your pastry, you *can* wrap it in clingfilm and keep it in the fridge while you prepare the filling, but it is by no means necessary. Unless otherwise stated in the recipe, you can make the pastry, fill it and immediately place it in the oven to bake. Because I use a mix of gluten-free flours (potato, corn, cassava) the pastry won't colour very much when baked. For this reason I suggest that you lightly brush the outside of the tart with rice milk before baking which will add a lovely golden hue.

White Soda Bread

Makes 1 loaf

—

450g/1lb gluten-free
    plain flour (ideally
    Doves Farm), plus
    extra for dusting
1 tsp bicarbonate of soda
¼ tsp xanthan gum
1 tsp caster sugar
1 tsp sea salt

For the soured milk
425ml/15fl oz rice milk
Juice of ½ lemon

A lovely allergy-friendly take on Irish soda bread, this is easy to make, with just a little bit of preparation in advance. Traditionally you would use buttermilk in the dough, but soured dairy-free milk works just as well. This bread is great served for breakfast, lunch or supper, so feel free to make it whenever you get the urge. It's best eaten fresh from the oven, however, as it doesn't lend itself to keeping.

You will need to make the soured milk a day in advance in order to let it sit. Begin by warming through the rice milk in a small saucepan, then remove from the heat and add the lemon juice. Cover and leave at room temperature overnight.

Preheat the oven to 230°C/450°F/gas mark 8 and lightly dust a baking sheet with flour.

Sift all the remaining ingredients into a large bowl and make a well in the centre. Pour most of the soured milk into the well, retaining about 50ml/1¾fl oz. Using your fingers, pull the flour and milk together until you have a soft, but not sticky, dough. If you think the dough is too dry, add a little more of the soured milk.

Once you have made the dough, turn it out onto a lightly floured work surface and shape it into a round loaf approximately 4cm/1½in thick. Cut a cross into the top of the bread, about 1cm/½in deep, and place on the prepared baking sheet.

Bake in the oven for 15 minutes, then reduce the temperature to 200°C/400°F/gas mark 6 and continue to bake for a further 30 minutes or until golden. The loaf will have a thick, crisp crust but feel heavy and solid to the touch. Remove from the oven and cool on a wire rack before serving.

Rye Soda Bread

Makes 1 small loaf

—

25ml/1fl oz rapeseed oil,
   plus extra for greasing
250g/9oz rye flour
   (ideally Doves Farm)
1 tsp bicarbonate of soda
2 tsp xanthan gum
A good pinch of sea salt
225ml/8fl oz rice milk
1 tbsp pumpkin seeds

*You will need a 450g/1lb
loaf tin for this recipe*

Bread is always a difficult thing to replace in the diet – especially when wheat, dairy, eggs and yeast are taken out of the equation. Yet there is nothing more pleasing than being able to rustle up a loaf, fresh and fragrant from the oven, ready to serve for breakfast or with a warming bowl of soup for lunch. Rye flour is naturally dense and contains a little gluten so can hold its own despite the lack of yeast; it has a sweet and nutty flavour (which the rapeseed oil enhances), making it wonderfully robust and particularly delicious. It is best served slightly warm, fresh from the oven, but it will keep for a few days and makes lovely toast. It also goes to perfection with smoked salmon, such as my Salmon Carpaccio with Caper Dressing or Hot-smoked Salmon Pâté (see pages 126 and 174).

Preheat the oven to 220°C/425°F/gas mark 7 and lightly grease the loaf tin.

In a large bowl, stir together the rye flour, bicarbonate of soda, xanthan gum and salt and make a well in the centre. Pour in the rice milk and rapeseed oil and stir together with a wooden spoon until the mixture pulls together into a soft and slightly tacky ball of dough.

Push the dough into the loaf tin, fitting it into the corners and levelling the top. Scatter over the pumpkin seeds, pushing down with the flat of your hand so that they become embedded in the dough. Using a sharp knife, make a cut, around 2.5cm/1in deep, running down the length of dough and then leave to stand somewhere warm for 30 minutes. (I recommend putting it in an airing cupboard or next to a radiator.)

Bake in the oven for 40–45 minutes or until crisp on the outside. Remove from the oven and turn out of the tin onto a wire rack to cool before cutting into wedges to serve.

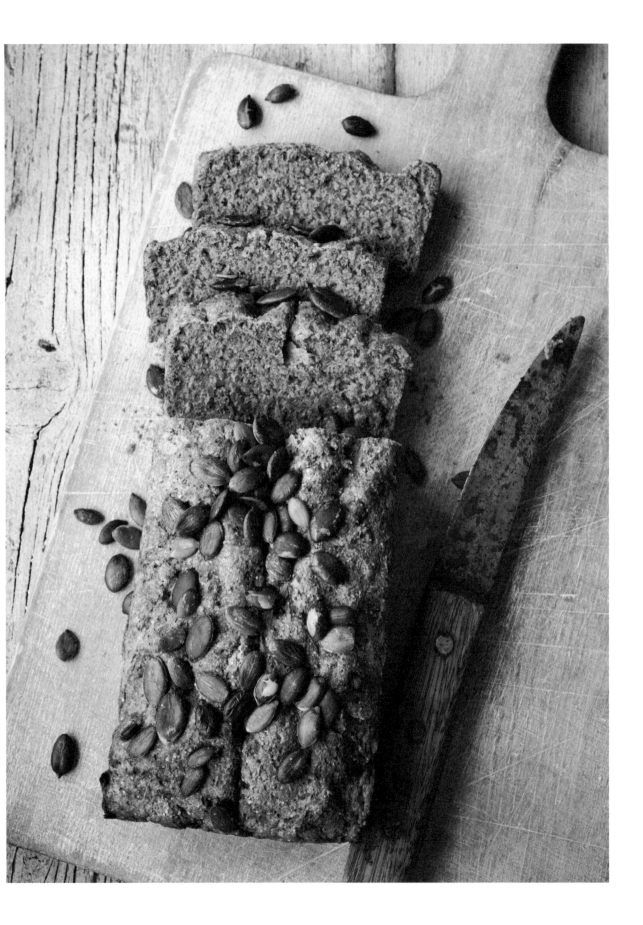

Flaxseed Bread

Makes 2 small loaves

—

500g/1lb 2oz gluten-free
    brown bread flour
    (ideally Doves Farm),
    plus extra for sprinkling
2 tsp bicarbonate of soda
50g/1¾oz golden
    caster sugar
1 tsp baking powder
2 tbsp ground flaxseeds
Good pinch of sea salt
85g/3¼oz Pure
    Sunflower Spread
    (dairy-free margarine),
    plus extra for greasing

For the soured milk
475ml/17fl oz rice milk
2 tbsp lemon juice

*You will need two 450g/
1lb loaf tins for this recipe*

These gorgeous little loaves are my interpretation of Irish wheaten bread (wholewheat soda bread). Traditionally made with wholewheat flour and buttermilk, this version uses a mix of brown rice flour, potato flour and ground flaxseeds bound together with soured rice milk. The result is a light and moist bread with a sweet and malty flavour, making it ideal for serving for breakfast or afternoon tea. I especially like it with pâté – you could try it with the Hot-smoked Salmon Pâté on page 174. The sweet/salty combination is a real favourite of mine.

First make the soured milk. Pour the rice milk into a jug or bowl, add the lemon juice and leave to stand while you prepare the other ingredients. (You may find that the rice milk will separate if left long enough; this is nothing to worry about as it will bind together again when mixed into the flour.)

Stir together the flour, bicarbonate of soda, sugar, baking powder, flaxseeds and salt in a large bowl. Cut the margarine into small chunks and add it to the bowl. Using your fingertips, rub in the margarine until the mixture resembles breadcrumbs.

Pour the soured milk over the crumb mixture and beat in with a wooden spoon until fully combined. Divide the mixture equally between the prepared loaf tins, smoothing over the top of each loaf with the back of the spoon. Sprinkle a little extra flour over the top and bake in the oven for 40 minutes or until golden brown and fragrant but not risen.

Remove the loaves from the oven, turn out of their tins and return to the oven, directly on the oven shelf, for a further 10 minutes. Place the loaves on a wire rack and allow to cool before serving.

Quinoa Bread

Makes 1 small loaf

—

125g/4½oz gluten-free
  plain flour (ideally
  Doves Farm), plus
  extra for dusting
125g/4½oz quinoa flour
¾ tsp bicarbonate of soda
½ tsp baking powder
A good pinch of sea salt
100g/3½oz Pure
  Sunflower Spread
  (dairy-free margarine)
1 tbsp runny honey

For the soured milk
250ml/9fl oz rice milk
2 tsp lemon juice

*You will need a 450g/1lb
loaf tin for this recipe*

*I am a huge fan of quinoa, with its mellow flavour and health-giving
properties; you can always find it in some form in my kitchen. Quinoa
flour works well in baking and tastes delicious made up into this bread.
The addition of a little margarine gives it an almost cakey texture, not
unlike brioche, which complements the slightly sweet flavour of the
quinoa. It's just right for breakfast or a light lunch or supper, served
with a salad, pâté or a bowl of soup.*

Preheat the oven to 180°C/350°F/gas mark 4 and lightly dust the loaf
tin with flour.

First make the soured milk. Pour the rice milk into a jug, add the
lemon juice and leave to stand for up to 1 hour. (You will see that the
rice milk separates quite distinctly, but don't panic as it will come back
together when you stir in the honey.)

Next, sift the plain flour and quinoa flour into a large bowl with the
bicarbonate of soda, baking powder and salt. Cut the margarine into
small cubes and lightly rub into the flour mixture – as though you were
making a crumble – until it becomes breadcrumb-like in consistency.

Stir the honey into the soured milk and pour this over the crumb
mixture. Stir together with a wooden spoon until combined (the
mixture will be quite liquid and a little lumpy) and then pour into
the prepared loaf tin.

Bake in the oven for around 45 minutes or until golden and fragrant
but not risen, then remove from the oven and carefully transfer from
the tin onto a wire rack to cool before serving.

Crusty White Loaf

Makes 1 loaf

—

450g/1lb gluten-free
   plain flour (ideally
   Doves Farm), plus
   extra for dusting
1 tsp bicarbonate of soda
2 tsp baking powder
3 tsp xanthan gum
A good pinch of sea salt
3 heaped tsp egg replacer
   (ideally Orgran) whisked
   with 6 tbsp water
175ml/6fl oz rice milk
1 tsp lemon juice
200ml/7fl oz sparkling
   water

*You will need a 450g/1lb
loaf tin for this recipe*

Allergy-friendly bread can be one of the hardest things to create; the lack of gluten, eggs and yeast makes it tricky to bake a loaf that can both rise and hold its shape. I promise you that this loaf will not disappoint, however. With a glorious crisp crust and just the right inner texture, it is a breeze to prepare and tastes equally good fresh from the oven or toasted the next day. You'll see when it bakes that it rises up brilliantly from its tin; this is due to the combination of sparkling water, bicarbonate of soda and lemon, which mimic the action of yeast but with none of the downsides for those who are intolerant to it. This truly is a failsafe recipe for bread – I love it and I hope you will too.

Preheat the oven to 200°C/400°F/gas mark 6 and lightly dust the loaf tin with flour.

Sift the flour, bicarbonate of soda, baking powder, xanthan gum and salt into a large bowl and stir together until blended. Pour in the egg replacer mixture, rice milk and lemon juice and, using a wooden spoon, mix everything together as much as you can – you will find the mixture is very dry and clumpy, which is as it should be.

Immediately pour over the sparkling water and mix together for a minute or so until the dough has pulled together. Now use your hands to lightly pull the mixture together, without kneading it, into one large ball of smooth dough – you will be able to feel how light and airy the dough is under your fingers. Resisting the urge to knead it, place the dough straight into the loaf tin, fitting it into the corners and then gently levelling the top with a spatula or the back of a spoon.

Bake in the oven for 45 minutes, by which time the loaf will have risen up out of the tin and turned a pale gold in colour with a crisp crust. Remove from the oven and transfer from the tin onto a wire rack, leaving to cool before cutting into slices.

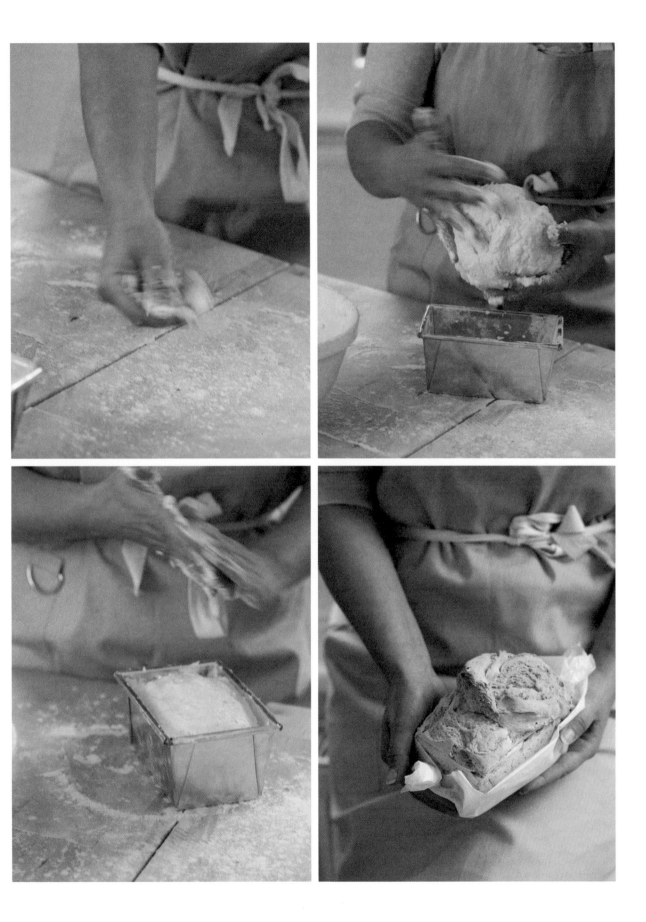

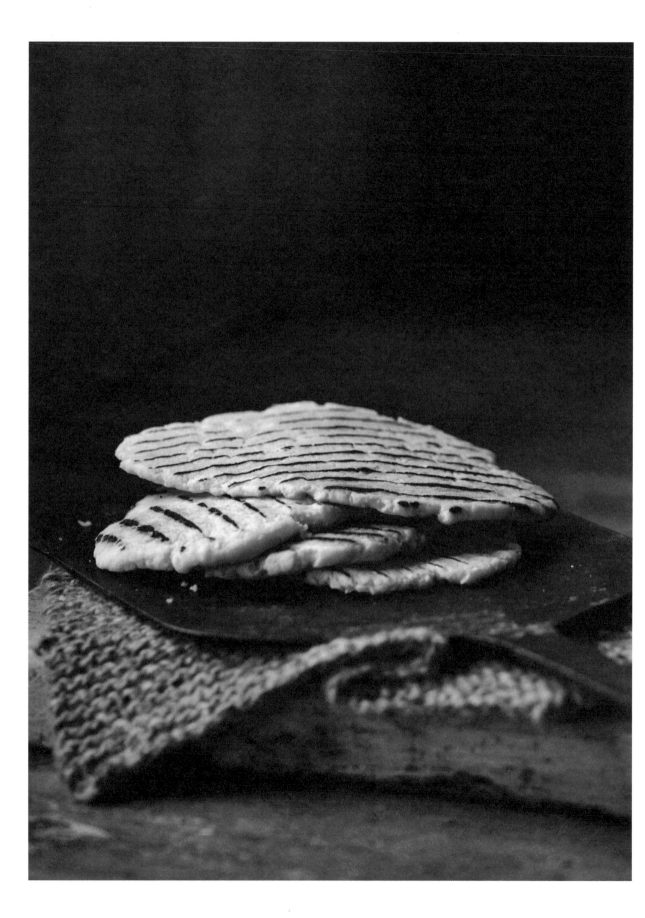

Flatbreads

Makes 2 flatbreads

—

110g/4oz gluten-free
   self-raising flour
   (ideally Doves Farm)
¼ tsp xanthan gum
A good pinch of sea salt
1 tbsp olive oil
4–6 tbsp warm water

Flatbreads, unleavened by yeast, are a staple food in many countries and nothing goes better with a platter of mezze, in my view, than these little breads with their smoky flavour and doughy texture. This is a very simple version of a classic flatbread which is quick and easy to throw together. Don't worry if the breads become a little charred in places when cooking; it will only add to the flavour. If you want to smarten these up, you can roll in a few roughly chopped herbs or scatter over some cumin seeds before cooking. Otherwise, they are lovely as they are.

Sift the flour into a large bowl with the xanthan gum and salt, making a well in the middle, then pour in the oil and water and mix into a stiff dough. (Add a little more water if the mixture is not coming together, bearing in mind that you don't want it to become sticky.) Pull the dough together with your hands and knead for around 2 minutes.

Divide the dough in half and roll into two balls. Place one ball of dough between two sheets of clingfilm and roll it out into an oval shape just under 1cm/½in thick, then remove the clingfilm and repeat with the second ball.

Meanwhile, heat a griddle pan or large non-stick frying pan until very hot. Lay the flatbreads in the pan and cook for about 3 minutes on each side or until browned. If you pan isn't big enough to hold both, cook them one at a time, keeping the first one warm in a clean tea towel until ready to eat. Serve immediately.

Corn Tortillas

Makes 10–12 tortillas

—

250g/9oz masa harina
(finely ground maize
flour)
A good pinch of sea salt
330ml/11½fl oz warm
water

Made with maize flour and hence naturally gluten-free, tortillas are an absolute blessing for those who are gluten-intolerant. They're quick to make, too, utterly delicious and so versatile. I serve them with falafel and my Greek Meatballs or Paprika Pepper Chicken (see pages 33, 93 and 83). I also fill them with salad and houmous or slices of avocado and cold grilled meat – the options are endless. Very finely ground maize flour, or masa harina, can be bought online or from specialist shops and some supermarkets (see Products and Stockists, page 231). It's well worth investing in as it makes by far the best tortillas. You can also make these using gluten-free plain flour and ¼ teaspoon of xanthan gum, but you'll need to an extra 100g/3½oz or so of flour in order to obtain the right consistency of dough.

Using a large bowl, mix together the masa harina, salt and water, stirring thoroughly until you have a smooth, thick batter, then cover and leave to stand for 15 minutes.

Check the consistency of the dough – it should feel soft and pliable but not sticky – and knead in a little extra water if necessary. Divide the dough into 10–12 portions and roll into balls each approximately 4cm/1½in in diameter, trying to make them as evenly round in shape as possible.

Heat a large griddle pan or non-stick frying pan until very hot. Meanwhile, place one of the tortilla balls between two sheets of clingfilm and roll or press into a circle around 3mm/⅛in thick. Alternatively, if you have one, use a tortilla press to flatten the dough.

Remove the clingfilm and dry-fry the tortilla in the hot pan for 15 seconds on one side, then turn it over and cook for a further 30 seconds on the other side. Turn the tortilla over again and wait a few seconds for it to puff up slightly. Once it has, remove from the pan and wrap in a clean tea towel while you roll out and cook the remaining tortillas. (You can roll out all the tortillas first, if you prefer, keeping the uncooked tortillas covered in another clean tea towel while you cook each of them.) Serve immediately or store, covered in clingfilm in an airtight container, and use to make wraps the next day.

Shortcrust Pastry

Makes 1 tart case

—

225g/8oz gluten-free
plain flour (ideally
Doves Farm)
½ tsp xanthan gum
60g/2oz Pure Sunflower
Spread (dairy-free
margarine), chilled
60g/2oz vegetable
shortening
2 tbsp caster sugar
(for sweet shortcrust
pastry only)

*You will need a 23cm/9in
tart tin with a removable
base for this recipe*

Light and biscuity in texture, this gluten-free shortcrust pastry provides the perfect base for a whole range of sweet and savoury tarts. What's more, it has two major advantages: you don't need to chill it and you don't need to bake it 'blind' before filling it. The addition of xanthan gum gives a smooth and glossy dough that is a breeze to use and tastes divine when cooked. I promise that once you have made this, your allergen-free cooking will be revolutionised and you'll never look back. I like to make my pastry in a food processor as it is so easy and effective, but if you don't have one you can make it by hand, following the instructions given below. The pastry won't colour very much when baked so I recommend brushing it with a little rice milk before baking to give it a gentle golden glow.

Sift the flour and xanthan gum into the bowl of a food processor, add the margarine and vegetable shortening and pulse until the mixture is of a breadcrumb-like consistency. Alternatively, place the ingredients in large bowl and rub together with your fingertips.

Tip in 2–3 tablespoons of cold water, a spoonful at a time and pulsing as you go (or stirring with a flat knife if making the pastry by hand) until the mixture begins to form a dough. If you are making sweet shortcrust pastry, add the caster sugar and pulse (or stir) for another minute before moving on to the next step.

Turn the pastry into a large bowl (or keep in the same bowl, if making it by hand) and, using your fingertips, pull together into a ball of dough. Knead gently for about 2 minutes or until smooth and elastic to the touch. Wrap the pastry in clingfilm and set aside or put in the fridge while you make the filling for the tart. (If you're making the pastry in advance, you can leave the pastry in the fridge for up to a week, removing it from the fridge and letting it come up to room temperature before rolling it out. It doesn't otherwise need to be chilled before using.)

Place the pastry between two large sheets of clingfilm (this makes rolling out gluten-free pastry so much easier) and roll it out into a circle slightly larger than the tart tin and no thinner than 3mm/⅛in. Peel off the uppermost sheet of clingfilm and carefully lay the pastry in the tin, gently pressing it into the sides. Fill any cracks or gaps with extra pastry, patted flat with your fingertips, and trim the edges. You are now ready to fill your tart case and bake in the oven.

Basic Biscuits

Makes 16–18 biscuits
Variations contain nuts
—

For the basic dough
125g/4½oz Pure
    Sunflower Spread
    (dairy-free margarine)
75g/3oz soft light brown
    sugar
150g/5oz gluten-free
    plain flour
    (ideally Doves Farm)
75g/3oz gluten-free
    self-raising flour
    (ideally Doves Farm)

For Cinnamon
2 tsp ground cinnamon
1 tbsp ground flaxseeds

For Custard Crunch
2 heaped tbsp dairy- and
    gluten-free custard powder

For Peanut Butter and
Chocolate
2 tbsp smooth peanut butter
50g/1¾oz dairy-free
    dark chocolate,
    roughly chopped,
    or chocolate nibs

For Pecan and Vanilla
100g/3½oz shelled pecan
    nuts, toasted and crushed
1 tsp vanilla extract

For Sultana and Spice
1 tsp mixed spice
50g/1¾oz sultanas
50g/1¾oz sunflower seeds

*You may need a 5cm/2in
diameter cookie cutter for
this recipe*

It's always worth having a good, basic biscuit recipe ready for those rainy days when you get the urge to bake. This simple dough can be adapted to make a number of delicious variations: Cinnamon, Custard Crunch, Peanut Butter and Chocolate, Pecan and Vanilla or Sultana and Spice. Whatever the flavour, these golden biscuits should be crisp and crunchy on the outside and softly chewy in the middle. They are best eaten on the day of baking, but can be stored in an airtight container for a further day.

Preheat the oven to 170°C/325°F/gas mark 3 and line two baking sheets with baking parchment. (Don't worry if you only have one baking sheet – just cook the biscuits in two batches.)

In a large bowl, cream together the margarine and sugar until pale and creamy. Sift in the flours, add the extra biscuit ingredients (if using) for one of the variations and mix together until fully combined – the mixture can be slightly clumpy. Then, using your hands, knead the mixture to form a loose dough.

Pinch off small amounts of the dough and, using the palms of your hands, roll into balls approximately 2.5cm/1in in diameter, then lay out on the baking sheets, spacing them evenly apart and adding 8–9 per sheet. Use the back of a fork to flatten the balls until they are roughly 1cm/½in thick – the biscuits will become rough around the edges, losing their smooth outline. Alternatively, place the dough between two sheets of clingfilm and roll out to the same thickness, then remove the clingfilm and cut into circles with the biscuit cutter before transferring to the baking sheets.

Bake in the oven for 15–17 minutes, switching the baking sheets between shelves after 7 minutes and rotating each sheet by 180 degrees, until lightly golden brown. Remove from the oven and transfer to a wire rack to cool.

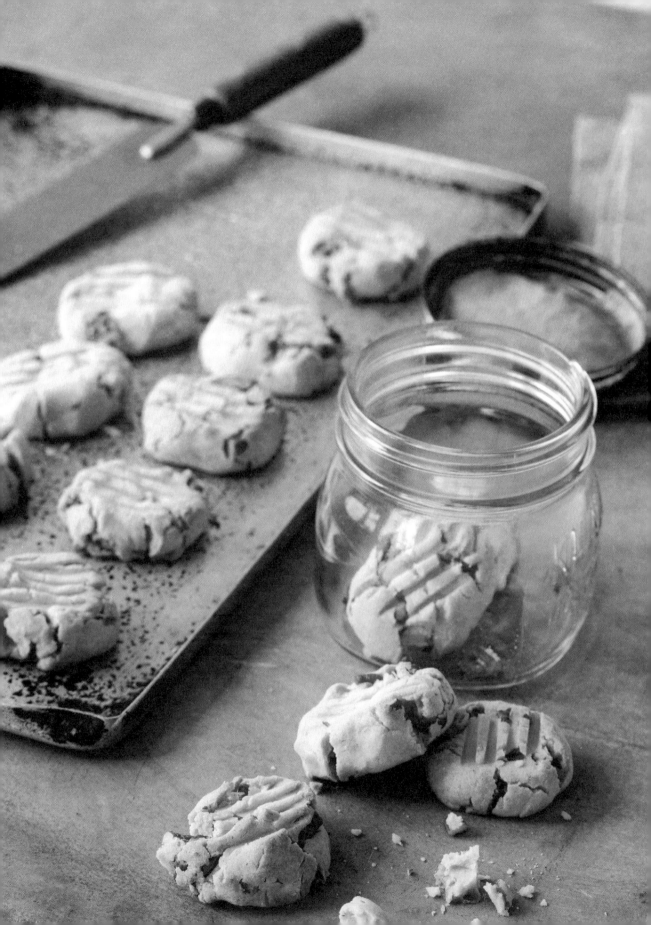

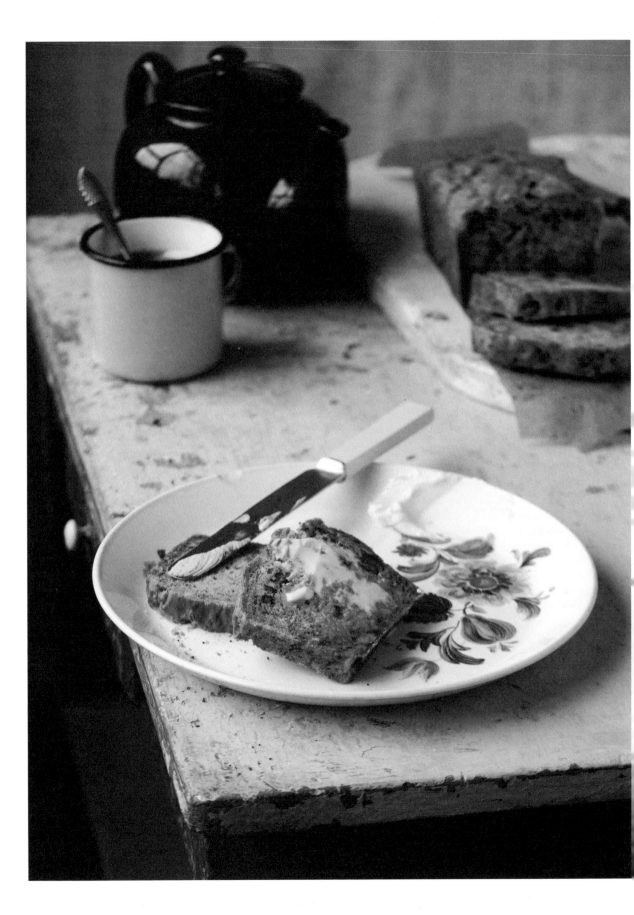

Banana Bread

Makes 1 loaf

—

100g/3½oz Pure
  Sunflower Spread
  (dairy-free margarine),
  plus extra for greasing
3 very ripe bananas
225g/8oz gluten-free
  self-raising flour
  (ideally Doves Farm)
125ml/4½fl oz agave
  syrup
½ tsp ground cinnamon
100g/3½oz shelled
  pecan nuts
2 heaped tsp egg replacer
  (ideally Orgran) whisked
  with 4 tbsp water
½ tsp bicarbonate
  of soda
1 tbsp warm water

*You will need a 900g/2lb
loaf tin for this recipe*

I love this recipe. It reminds me of lazy days spent on the beach, windswept and salty, wrapped in a towel and clutching a thick slice of banana bread in my hands. It makes a delicious afternoon treat, a favourite for a rainy day and indispensable for a picnic. The beauty of this recipe is that you can make it all in the food processor with minimum effort, allowing you to run up a sumptuous banana loaf whenever the whim takes you. This bread is best served on the day you make it, but still tastes good, lightly toasted and buttered, a couple of days later. Stored in an airtight container, it will last for up to four days.

Preheat the oven to 180°C/350°F/gas mark 4, then lightly grease the loaf tin and line the base and sides with baking parchment.

Peel and roughly chop the bananas and add to a food processor with the margarine, flour, agave syrup, cinnamon, pecan nuts and egg replacer mixture. Mix together the bicarbonate of soda with the warm water (the two will foam together on contact) and tip into the food processor, then pulse until you have a thick and creamy batter.

Alternatively you can make the batter by hand. First mash the bananas into a smooth purée in a large bowl. Add the margarine, agave syrup and egg replacer mixture and stir together, then add the flour, pecan nuts and cinnamon and beat until you have a smooth batter. Mix together the bicarbonate of soda and warm water and then pour into the batter and beat together quickly.

Pour the batter into the prepared loaf tin, levelling the top with a spatula or the back of a spoon, then bake in the oven for 25–30 minutes or until risen, golden brown and firm to a light touch. Allow to cool in the tin for 10 minutes before turning out onto a wire rack to finish cooling.

Products and Stockists

Shopping can seem a daunting task when first looking for allergy- or intolerance-friendly products. By far the best place to go is your local health-food shop, where you will be able to ask detailed questions about the products on offer and how they are used. I recommend finding a good one locally and building a relationship with the owners; you will be amazed at the lengths people will go to when they genuinely care about the products they supply. Saying that, there are times when convenience dictates a trip to the supermarket, and fortunately most supermarkets now stock a large range of allergy-friendly foods and at reasonable prices. Another way to shop is via the internet, where a growing number of 'supermarkets' offer a vast array of allergen-free products. Shopping online, while not instant, does have the advantage of a huge degree of choice with the convenience of having the goods delivered straight to your door.

Like all enthusiastic cooks, I love a well-stocked pantry and being intolerance-friendly doesn't make mine any less full. You will be pleasantly surprised at how many 'true' foods you can eat and dazzled at the number of allergy- and intolerance-friendly products on the market. Over the years, I have tried them all and found that some far surpass others, so much so that I tend not to use anything else. A comprehensive list of naturally intolerance-friendly ingredients for your storecupboard is given in 'The Intolerant Kitchen' (see page 12), all of which are widely available from health-food shops and big supermarkets. This section is devoted to my storecupboard essentials – a list of those products that I rate the most highly and the website addresses of the main stockists that provide them. I recommend stocking up on a good supply of these, so that you always have some to hand. While it may be easy to nip to the local shop for a carton of cow's milk or a standard loaf of bread, the allergen-free varieties aren't always so easy to come by.

It is worth noting that new products are continually appearing and it is good to experiment with them yourself to find out which ones you like best. This list could keep growing and reflects the ingredients used in this book, but for now these are, in my opinion, the best allergy- and intolerance-friendly products currently available.

Dairy Substitutes

For more on dairy-free milks, fats and oils, see 'The Intolerant Kitchen' (pages 12–21).

Milk and Cream

Ecomil Almond Milk

A good milk substitute for baking and in sauces for curries, this is also delicious for pouring over cereal, especially granola or muesli; it uses agave syrup as a sweetener.
www.goodnessdirect.co.uk
www.waitrose.co.uk

Ecomil Almond Milk Powder

A powdered version of their almond milk with no added sweetener. The chief benefit of using powdered milk is that you can control the degree of thickness of the liquid. It is also very handy for making ice cream.
www.goodnessdirect.co.uk

Ecomil Hazelnut Milk

Again, a good milk substitute for baking, with a thick and creamy texture and a sweet and subtle hazelnut taste.
www.goodnessdirect.co.uk
www.waitrose.co.uk

Oatly Chocolate Milk

A version of Oatly Milk with the addition of cocoa powder and sugar, this delicious and creamy milk is perfect for making hot chocolate, custard or summertime milkshakes.
www.goodnessdirect.co.uk
www.sainsburys.co.uk
www.waitrose.co.uk

Oatly Oat Cream

A rich and velvety alternative to cream, this is perfect for pouring over puddings, and ideal for use in baking, cream-based dishes and sauces.
www.goodnessdirect.co.uk
www.waitrose.com

Oatly Oat Milk

This oat milk is light and creamy, making it good for adding to tea or coffee, pouring over cereal or for using to make ice cream. Because it is heat stable, it is suitable for using in cooking and baking, its neutral flavour making it perfect for adding to sauces.
www.goodnessdirect.co.uk
www.sainsburys.co.uk
www.waitrose.com

Rice Dream Rice Milk

Good for use in baking and sauces, this is also my milk of choice for pouring over cereals and, more importantly, adding to tea or coffee.
www.goodnessdirect.co.uk
www.sainsburys.co.uk
www.waitrose.com

Butter

Biona Sunflower Margarine

A good-quality trans-fat-free margarine. The texture is a little grainier than Pure Sunflower Spread and it can become a little oily when used in large quantities for cooking (as in baking), but it has a good flavour nonetheless. Ideal for making sauces or simply to spread on bread.
www.goodnessdirect.co.uk

Biona Organic Coconut Oil

With a creamy, sweet and strong flavour, coconut oil reacts in much the same way as butter when heated, making it ideal for use in cooking, especially baking. Coconut oil is a naturally saturated and completely trans-fat-free oil that becomes a solid when stored at room temperature.
www.goodnessdirect.co.uk

Pure Sunflower Spread

A trans-fat-free margarine made from sunflower oil, this is the best substitute for butter on the market. With a rich yellow colour, it acts in

much the same way as butter when cooked at medium temperatures.
www.goodnessdirect.co.uk
www.sainsburys.co.uk
www.waitrose.com

Rapeseed oil – Clearspring / Farrington's Mellow Yellow/Hillfarm

Rapeseed oil is a good substitute for butter in all types of cooking, including roasting, frying and baking.
www.goodnessdirect.co.uk
www.sainsburys.co.uk
www.waitrose.co.uk

Egg Substitutes

For more on the use of apple purée and ground flaxseeds as a substitute for eggs, see 'The Intolerant Kitchen' (pages 15–16).

Clearspring Organic Apple Fruit Purée

This 100 per cent fruit purée is great to have as a standby in your storecupboard for use as an egg replacement, adding a light and fruity flavour to your baking.
www.goodnessdirect.co.uk
www.waitrose.co.uk

Energ-G Egg Replacer

Similar to Orgran in its ingredients, this is a good-quality egg replacer that works well in cakes, breads, biscuits and other baking.
www.ener-g.com
www.goodnessdirect.co.uk

Life Free From Egg Free Mayonnaise

This is the only egg-, dairy- and soya-free mayonnaise I have been able to find and it just happens to be wonderful. It has a smooth, velvety texture and works well as a dressing, dip or marinade.
www.frylight.co.uk
www.waitrose.co.uk

Orgran No Egg Natural Egg Replacer

The best egg-, dairy-, soya- and yeast-free egg replacer on the market. Although not ideal for making scrambled eggs (!), it does work very well in cakes, breads and biscuits.
www.goodnessdirect.co.uk

Prewetts Ground Flaxseed

Ground flaxseeds work best as a binder (when mixed with water) and so are ideal for using as an egg substitute, especially in muffins and cakes.
www.goodnessdirect.co.uk

Gluten-Free Basics

Flour

For more on gluten-free flours, see 'The Intolerant Kitchen' (page 16).

Doves Farm Gluten Free Brown Bread Flour

I cannot recommend Doves Farm flours highly enough; they are essential for the intolerance-friendly kitchen. This bread flour uses a combination of rice, tapioca, sarrasin, carob, sugar beet fibre and xanthan gum to create a light, brown bread flour, ideal for allergy-free brown loaves.
www.dovesfarm.co.uk
www.goodnessdirect.co.uk
www.sainsburys.co.uk

Doves Farm Gluten Free Plain Flour

Made from a combination of cassava, potato and rice flours, this plain flour acts as the perfect all-rounder for bread, pastry, sauces and many other recipes using flour.
www.dovesfarm.co.uk
www.goodnessdirect.co.uk
www.sainsburys.co.uk
www.waitrose.co.uk

Doves Farm Gluten Free Self-Raising Flour
As with all Doves Farm flours, I cannot recommend this highly enough. Ideal for all baking recipes, it contains just the right blend of flours plus a little extra xanthan gum to create perfectly textured cakes and bread.
www.dovesfarm.co.uk
www.goodnessdirect.co.uk
www.sainsburys.co.uk
www.waitrose.co.uk

Goodness Organic Quinoa Flour
A light and grainy flour with a distinctive flavour, this produces a good loaf of bread when mixed with other, smoother, gluten-free flours.
www.goodnessdirect.co.uk

Masa harina
This traditional Mexican flour, used for making tortillas and tamales, is made from very finely ground maize flour and needs only a little water to form it into a rich dough; an absolute 'must have' for your storecupboard. For suppliers, visit:
www.mexgrocer.co.uk
www.sainsburys.co.uk

Cereals

Nairn's Gluten Free Real Porridge Oats
Produced in a strictly controlled, dedicated gluten-free environment, Nairn's gluten-free oats are ideal for using in any baking recipe and are delicious made for breakfast, a little pouring of rice milk and some brown sugar as their accompaniment.
www.goodnessdirect.co.uk
www.sainsburys.co.uk
www.waitrose.co.uk

Doves Farm Gluten Free Cornflakes
Another product from the Doves Farm collection, this cereal has all the flavour and crunch of cornflakes without the added barley which is so common in other brands. I recommend them for use in baking and simply to eat with a pouring of your favourite dairy-free milk.
www.dovesfarm.co.uk
www.sainsburys.co.uk
www.waitrose.co.uk
www.goodnessdirect.co.uk

Bread

Although the market for wheat-free breads grows each year, there is still concern about the number of additives they contain and there remains little choice in the range of wheat- and yeast-free bread. Below you will find my list of the best wheat- and yeast-free breads available. You can purchase one or two of these from some supermarkets but the rest are available online.

Artisan Bread Organic
This incredible bakery makes organic, wheat-, gluten- and yeast-free breads and then delivers them fresh to your door. Made from natural ingredients and freshly milled flours, including buckwheat, pea, quinoa, rice and rye, they are an absolute dream. I highly recommend the quinoa bread, which has a wonderful texture and flavour. Plus, you can place a bulk order and then freeze the loaves ready to defrost whenever you require one.
www.artisanbread-abo.com

Biona Organic Rye Bread
Biona is a good-quality brand and with a variety of long-life, yeast-free rye breads (including linseed, hemp and pumpkin seed). A naturally wheat-free loaf, it is delicious toasted but equally tasty for an open sandwich.
www.goodnessdirect.co.uk
www.waitrose.co.uk

Ener-G Rice Loaf
A gluten- and yeast-free pre-sliced loaf made
entirely from rice. Although I would advocate
making your own bread, it pays to have a few
back-up loaves tucked away in your pantry or
freezer. This particular one comes sealed in
a vacuum pack and so has a long shelf life; it makes
great toast and is also very useful for making
breadcrumbs. I wouldn't, however, recommend
eating it straight from the packet.
www.goodnessdirect.co.uk

The Village Bakery Organic Rye Bread
This is a rich and dense wheat-free bread that is
made without yeast. With a delicious flavour, it
makes lovely sandwiches and toasts beautifully
too. I always ensure I have a loaf of this on hand
for breakfast, lunch and impromptu tea and toast!
www.village-bakery.com
www.waitrose.co.uk

Pasta

Doves Farm Gluten Free Pasta
A lovely, light golden pasta with a nice smooth
texture. The Doves Farm range of spaghetti and
pasta is among the best available. You would be
hard pressed to tell these apart from good-quality
wheat-based pasta, and they cook in very much
the same way, making them ideal for nearly all
dishes using standard pasta.
www.dovesfarm.co.uk
www.sainsburys.co.uk
www.waitrose.co.uk

Rizopia Brown Rice Pasta
Rizopia is a specialist brand of gluten-free
pasta and spaghetti made entirely from brown
rice. These have a slightly denser texture than
corn-based pasta but a great flavour nonetheless,
making them one of the closest-tasting things
to 'real' pasta currently on the market.
www.rizopia.com
www.waitrose.co.uk

Salute
By far the best gluten-free pasta on the market,
this Italian-made, maize- and rice-based pasta
has a wonderful texture and a taste that beats
its wheat-based counterpart hands down!
I really recommend this for any pasta dish
you may want to make; it is truly delicious.
www.waitrose.co.uk

Baking Aids

*For more on intolerance-friendly baking aids,
see 'The Intolerant Kitchen' (page 20).*

Baking powder – Allergycare/Doves Farm/Dr Oetker
Gluten-free baking powder is a must-have
for all your baking.
www.dovesfarm.co.uk
www.goodnessdirect.co.uk
www.sainsburys.co.uk

Xanthan gum
This is an essential binding ingredient for
allergy-friendly baking. For suppliers, visit:
www.dovesfarm.co.uk
www.goodnessdirect.co.uk
www.sainsburys.co.uk
www.waitrose.co.uk

Sweet Extras

Agave syrup
This is a naturally sweet syrup made from
juice obtained from the agave plant. It is
sweeter than honey but not quite as sweet as
golden syrup. With a very slow sugar release,
it is much better for you than real syrup and
is ideal for baking with, as it adds a wonderful
gooey texture to cakes and puddings.
For suppliers, visit:
www.goodnessdirect.co.uk
www.sainsburys.co.uk
www.waitrose.co.uk

All Natural Custard Powder

A custard powder made from natural ingredients, it can be made up with any dairy-free milk and used as a base for ice creams or in biscuits to add a creamy, vanilla flavour.
www.goodnessdirect.co.uk
www.sainsburys.co.uk

Biona Almond Butter

This almond butter is made from lightly roasted batches of whole almonds, with no added sugar or salt. It is wonderful in homemade biscuits or granola bars, or you can spread it on toast for a delicious breakfast or snack.
www.goodnessdirect.co.uk

Green & Black's Cocoa Powder

This dark chocolate powder has a wonderfully intense flavour. I use it in baking and other puddings, as well as whisking it together with almond milk and a little agave syrup for a delicious hot chocolate.
www.goodnessdirect.co.uk
www.sainsburys.co.uk
www.waitrose.co.uk

Montezuma's Dark Chocolate

Montezuma makes a range of dark dairy- and soy-free chocolates, all of which are delicious. They are ideal for having on hand to bake with or just to nibble on when you get the urge!
www.goodnessdirect.co.uk
www.waitrose.co.uk

Savoury Extras

Colman's Mustard Powder

Made from grinding brown and white mustard seeds, this mustard powder is a handy storecupboard staple. You simply mix it with equal amounts of water to create a pungent condiment for adding to dressings, sauces and sandwiches. Please note that the ready-made version of this product contains wheat flour and so is not suitable for allergy-sufferers; only the mustard powder itself is gluten-free.
www.sainsburys.co.uk
www.waitrose.co.uk

Musk's Gluten Free Sausages

Unlike most gluten-free sausages, these are free from both gluten and egg. Made from good-quality pork and containing cooked rice as a binder, they're ideal for using in stews or as the basis for a classic sausage and mash.
www.sainsburys.co.uk
www.waitrose.co.uk

Allergy-Friendly Stocks

Chicken stock – Sainsbury's Signature/ Waitrose Cooks' Ingredients

These tubs and packets of chicken stock (fresh and long-life) are so handy to have around and have a delicious savoury flavour. The long-life is ideal for keeping in your cupboard, while the fresh version freezes really well, ready to be taken out and used in soups, stews, tagines or for cooking grains.
www.sainsburys.co.uk
www.waitrose.co.uk

Kallo Yeast Free Vegetable Stock

A storecupboard essential, this is available in cubes or as a powder.
www.goodnessdirect.co.uk
www.sainsburys.co.uk

Marigold Swiss Vegetable Vegan Bouillon Powder

Marigold bouillon powders have a great flavour as well as being among the few gluten-, dairy- and yeast-free stock powders on the market. This one is very simple to use and is handy for a variety of recipes – a storecupboard essential.
www.sainsburys.co.uk

Index

Acknowledgements

I am incredibly grateful to all of the people who have worked so hard to make this the book I truly wanted it to be, and whose faith and vision have helped to make it what it is.

Enormous thanks to Rosemary Scoular for her belief in me and brilliance in all matters; equal thanks to Wendy Millyard whose positivity and enthusiasm have been priceless. Thanks to all the team at Harper Collins for making my first publishing experience such a pleasure. Extra special thanks to Lizzy Gray for understanding exactly what I wanted to create and for having the talent and skill to produce it. A huge thank you to Myfanwy Vernon-Hunt for her eye for the beautiful detail and for liking all the things I like; and to George Atsiaris for her patience, editorial skills and brilliant hard work.

I couldn't have been luckier than getting to work with Jan Baldwin (and her team), whose exquisite photography, elegance and talent was so inspiring. Enormous thanks to food stylist extraordinare Joss Herd, who is, quite literally, a joy to behold and whose exceptional skills made the shoot a fortnight of delight. Everyone should have a Joss and Jan in their lives. Thanks also to Kate Parker for her excellent copyediting, Val McArthur for her kitchen skills, and Liz Belton and Jo Harris for their elegant taste in props. I am grateful, too, to Petra Börner for creating what I consider to be the most beautiful illustrations in the world.

Finally, thank you to my friends and family for their unstinting love, support and taste-testing. For my mum and dad who brought me up in a house filled with joyful cooking and enthusiasm for food; I couldn't have found my way so easily without that. For Miranda, especially, whose belief in me and whose drive and passion deserve a world of my thanks.

Last, but never least, thank you to my Patrick, for his love, kindness, humour and excellent appetite.

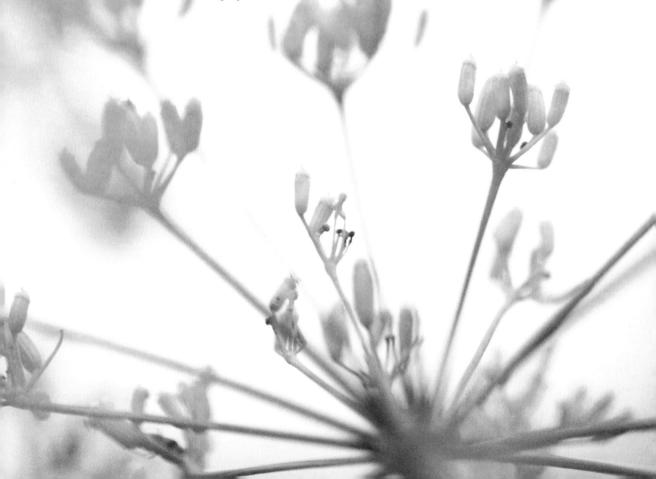

First published in 2012 by Collins,
an imprint of HarperCollins*Publishers*

77–85 Fulham Palace Road
Hammersmith
London, W6 8JB
www.harpercollins.co.uk

10 9 8 7 6 5 4 3 2 1

A catalogue record of this book is available from the British Library

ISBN 978-0-00-744864-7

Printed and bound in China by South China Printing Company Ltd

Food stylists – Joss Herd and Val McArthur
Prop stylists – Liz Belton and Jo Harris